Memoirs from my Mended Heart

There is life after heart surgery

Robert John Roberts

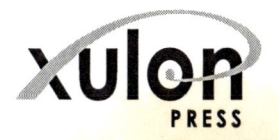

xulon PRESS

Copyright © 2008 by Robert John Roberts

Memoirs from my Mended Heart
There is life after heart surgery
by Robert John Roberts

Printed in the United States of America

ISBN 978-1-60477-564-8

All rights reserved solely by the author. The author guarantees all contents are original and do not infringe upon the legal rights of any other person or work. No part of this book may be reproduced in any form without the permission of the author. The views expressed in this book are not necessarily those of the publisher.

Unless otherwise indicated, Bible quotations are taken from The Authorized King James Version. Copyright © 1909 by Oxford University Press, Inc.

www.xulonpress.com

Preface

Faulkner, a celebrated Southern literary genius, put it best when he encouraged writers to "write about what you know." Langston Hughes was advised "to go home and write a page, but let that page come out of you." I have discovered in my short life that fact is often more compelling than fiction. The pages that follow contain facts that I know to be true and I experienced in my life. I can validate what I say because I lived through this and experienced all the things I wrote myself. Note to the analytical mind: this memoir was penned in stream of consciousness style. To the average reader this simply means my story was penned as I saw it unfold in my mind. Sometimes it was confusing, but nonetheless it was the way I had to live through a bewildering time in my life.

There is nothing I despise more than to waste my valuable time reading a book with a misleading forward.

Therefore, this is the account of my journey to death's door twice in 47 short days. If this chronicle helps one soul who is suffering along life's way, it will have been well worth my efforts. This undertaking has already been very therapeutic and cathartic for me. Putting my feelings, emotions, and struggles on paper has afforded me an outlet I could find nowhere else. The long and short of it is that I miraculously survived an aortic dissection and a category F4 tornado along with several other near death experiences after I thought about it. It is no mystery why God allowed me to live through these two life threatening events; my life was spared to declare the love, mercy, goodness, provision, and sovereignty of God. If you want to know more, read on. If you want to put this book down, go ahead. Either way, you have been informed of what is ahead.

For Miranda and Hines,
You both keep my heart beating strong.

There is life after heart surgery...

It was lightly misting that bleak, cold morning in February when Miranda left for work. She was wearing a bright yellow rain jacket. I still remember the melodic sound of synthetic fabric brushing against itself as she walked down our hall and out the back door, arms swinging at her sides. She wore this same jacket until I regained consciousness because the doctors told her I may or may not recognize her. That is true love. It was three days before I would fully recognize her after that morning. Yellow has long been one of my favorite colors. It is a vibrant color that is bright, happy, and full of life. But no yellow has ever brought a smile to my face the way that yellow jacket did as the emergency team rounded the corner of that long empty hallway. The morphine I had been given was in full effect, and I was loaded! There is a good reason why that medicine is not sold over the counter. High as a Georgia pine, I asked the paramedics if there was a woman in a yellow jacket heading towards us or if there was in fact some major chicanery going on in my mind. Never missing a step, the paramedics just kept steadily rolling me to my next destination.

My new friend whom I got to know on the ambulance ride said, "Yeah John, you're not hallucinating. By the way she is headed towards us it looks like you are the person she is looking for." The distance between us quickly closed, and soon her hand was in mine. All I asked God that day was to see my wife before I was put under for surgery. He not only granted my request but also allowed Miranda to be the first person I saw after I was rolled out of the ambulance. As my stretcher sped down the hall, we were the only two people on the planet. My life was hanging in the balance. My body wanted to give up, but my heart just wouldn't quit. When Miranda gripped my hand, I knew everything was going to be fine.

Joe E. Lewis once said, "You only live once, but if you work it right, once is enough." We should savor each day as though it could be our last because it very well could be.

Let us take a stroll through the corridors of my life heretofore. I have faced many obstacles in my short 28 years on this Earth. Death has even pulled my ticket a few times; it just hasn't been punched... yet. From the first time up to this most recent brush, there is one common thread; one carries very vivid memories of a near death experience. When we experience a stressful situation in life, the memory of the event often becomes extremely amplified. The most minute parts of the experience appear like HDTV, usually for the rest of one's life. The first time I ever remember, remember being the operative word, realizing that I was not immortal was on a Wednesday night around six o'clock. My parents were in our house getting ready to go to prayer meeting. I was in my front yard with my pellet gun mindlessly taking target practice as any little boy does at anything and everything. There was a brush pile smoldering in our front yard. I can still remember the scent of the pine limbs as they burned. There was one solid log still burning in the ashes. I vividly remember thinking that my gun could easily pierce the smoking twig. I closed one eye, took careful aim, gently exhaled the air in my lungs, and pulled the trigger. Chuuhhhh and the bullet was gone from the barrel. Instantly, I knew something was wrong. Something exploded in my mouth. I put my hand in front of my mouth and spat. Out came my front tooth in several pieces, along with the pellet which I had just fired from the air rifle. I still have that pellet. Thank God it was just a tooth I lost. It could have been my eye which was hit. Even worse, the shott could have penetrated my eye and entered my brain.

Not long after that little mishap, my Dad and I got caught in a severe thunderstorm over the mountains in North Georgia in his Cessna 170-A. One minute it was a clear, sunny day, and the next we were in the middle of a severe thunderstorm. Several times I glanced out my window to see tree tops feet below our landing gear through the pouring rain.

We were within a hair's breadth of smashing into an Appalachian mountain top. Dad was doing as best he could under the circumstances, but he needed my help. He pleaded with me to help him watch for the peaks. I was almost crying with my eyes closed tightly by this time. I didn't want to see the crash landing. One rule even green pilots know is that you don't fly in the mountains in bad weather. It can only lead to one thing, disaster.

My Dad had logged well over 2000 hours as a seasoned private pilot. I had never seen him even remotely nervous in his plane until that day. Looking back, I know he was more concerned for my safety than he was his own. Somehow through the storm he spotted a water tower with a red and white checker board pattern painted on it. It was one of the prettiest sights I had ever seen from the air. We didn't know it at the time, but we were flying over an Army Ranger Base that had a short runway nestled between rows of helicopters. By this point we were both ready to put the Cessna down on *Terra Firma*. Dad simply said, "Brace yourself John, I'm gonna put her on the ground. This may be a hard landing." With those words I witnessed the most graceful emergency landing I have ever seen.

Thank God this was before 9/11, or we may have been shot on site after our miraculous touchdown. As we taxied up to the only hanger, we were greeted by some men in camouflage, wielding assault rifles, and they looked like they were loaded for bear. A fire truck and ambulance soon appeared with a not so happy Colonel Brown. He curtly wanted to know our business, departure, destination, and how on earth we landed on his helicopter landing zone. The only thing the Rangers saw was a plane dropping out of the sky sideways, in order to quickly descending, and disappear behind the tree line. Needless to say we cut it close that day, so close that when we rolled the old Cessna around to tie her down, I pulled a pine tree branch from in between the strut and wheel pan.

I never had a traffic accident in my teenage years, but I was caught speeding three times before I turned eighteen. Each time I was stopped, it was for traveling in excess of 80 miles per hour. I have always wondered if thanking the officer for looking out for my safety resulted in a break on the ticket and my not losing my license. Life is full of irony. The officer who wrote all my speeding tickets lives on the rural mail route I currently serve. It is amazing how I ever made it to my eighteenth birthday considering my lead foot. I often ponder how many times I flirted with death all those times when there was no state trooper on the highway to catch me.

During my senior year of high school, I ate a not so tasty dirt sandwich on a Honda CR125 dirt bike. My cousin and I had been riding all afternoon. I had just spoken with my mom and dad as they headed out for an afternoon bicycle ride. The last thing my father told me was, "Son, don't do anything foolish to get hurt." Ty decided to call it a day while I lined up for one more evil jump across our driveway. I shifted through second and pinned the throttle in third as I hit the jump. I can still remember looking over at the gravel road, parallel to the ditch I had just launched out of, and thinking to myself, "Boy. This is gonna leave a mark." I distinctly remember hearing dad's words run through my mind, "don't do anything foolish." What I did was above and beyond foolish; it was plain stupid. I grew up riding street bikes, not dirt bikes. I was under the impression that because I had been on motorcycles for many years, I was an experienced rider. I quickly discovered experience on a street bike does not make one a seasoned motocross rider.

Dad always told me that if I ever went down on a bike, to try to tuck and roll. This advice proved invaluable. I grabbed the mouth guard on my helmet in that split second one realizes this is the point of no return and pulled my head down into my chest with all the force I could muster. Being at the point in a jump when I was almost floating, I managed to perform a half front flip. My orthopedic surgeon told me this was a smart move because had I impacted on my feet, I would have probably shattered both my legs from such a high fall. We estimated I was at least twenty feet in the air when I came off the motorcycle. I escaped serious injury, and limped away with a fractured pelvis, broken collar bone, and some major bruises.

One injury was a deep contusion to my heart. This resulted in six weeks being spent sitting in a wheelchair, which could have just as easily turned into a lifetime had God not had His hand upon my landing in the bottom of that ditch. About two weeks earlier, Christopher Reeve, Superman no less, had taken a header off of a horse which resulted in permanent paralysis. My mom reminded me of this fact more than once as I was confined to my wheelchair. I always thanked God my parents were not home when I crashed and burned because if they had seen my limp body lying in the bottom of the ditch, they would have both probably suffered heart attacks simultaneously. The only lasting result of the crash was arthritis at an early age. For several years after the accident when I would complain of the aches, my Dad simply repeated two words, twice: "Disobedience son, disobedience son." In that wheelchair I learned a lot about myself and especially whom I could depend on in hard times.

The accident happened the week before Spring Break. All my friends were going to Panama City Beach for the last time during Senior year. Some offered to take me with them, but I didn't want to be a burden on anyone, and I was still in a considerable amount of pain at that point. There was one person whom I came to think very highly of during those six weeks. Bruce Williams would come over every day after school and hang out with me. He was one of the few friends I had who didn't forget about me. I will be eternally grateful to him for the empathy he showed me as I recovered. He came to be the only person my mom would let me leave the house with as I improved enough to get out in a vehicle. She said he looked like a safe driver. I always wondered if it was because he drove a four-door Caprice.

The Bible bears out the fact in Matthew 18:10 that we have guardian angels: "Take heed that ye despise not one of these little ones; for I say unto you, That in heaven their angels do always behold the face of my Father which is in heaven." Needless to say, I am thankful God gave me a swift guardian angel. I may even have two. A slothful spirit probably would not have worked for longevity in my case. In all these situations and circumstances I was always thankful God spared my life, as well as my physical health. However, I never truly appreciated my infirmities, and especially not my tribulations, in a Biblical sense. I never asked God what, if anything, He wanted me to learn during any of these brushes with my mortality. I was just glad to escape unscathed. Then, on February 3rd, 2005, I was forced to face my mortality in the most surreal way I could ever dream or imagine. As I have already said, fact is sometimes stranger than fiction.

January 29. Let us begin where I initially heard death's cold hand rapping at my door. On a Sunday, night during youth group at church, I experienced a searing white hot pain in the middle of my chest. All the muscles and tendons in my chest cavity felt as if they were slowly being ripped in half. After surgery, nurses always ask; what is your pain level, one being mild and ten being unbearable. Well the dirt bike wreck hurt pretty bad, but this pain was literally off the scale. It was real. There is really no way to put into words the pain I felt. Unless you have ever been privileged to live through an aortic dissection or had a full grown elephant stand on your chest and jump up and down simply use your imagination. Trust me when I say it was excruciating! In the back of my mind something told me, you need to get to the hospital, John. I ignored that little voice and attributed the feeling, if one could refer to it as such, to a pulled muscle or a wicked case of indigestion.

Pause for personal background information. I was born with a bicuspid aortic valve. Simply put, my aortic valve which normally looks like a Mercedes-Benz emblem was missing one of the leaves. A normal valve completely seals after the heart beats. A bicuspid valve cannot seal, thus allowing a small amount of blood to backwash into the heart each time it beats. This produces a subtle shish, or murmur, which identifies the problem. This is a common heart defect. Many people go for years and never even know they have one. My mother was 41 before they found hers, and I was eleven before mine surfaced in a routine physical. When Dr. Merritt carefully listened to my heart, he noticed the ever so slight shish of my valve. It required no special medication. I was only restricted from heavy lifting and full contact sports. This suited me just fine because I always enjoyed tennis more than football anyway.

While listening to our youth pastor's devotional to our youth group, I became light headed and extremely dizzy. The feeling intensified so that I thought I may pass out. This was very strange to me because I have never passed out from anything, even to this day. The possibility of a heart attack began racing in my mind like a greyhound chasing the little rabbit on the track. But I had never heard of a twenty-eight-year-old dying of a heart attack. I quickly reasoned. Surely that was not what is happening to me. Immediately I dismissed such a serious notion from my mind. Random advice: Never dismiss any possibility in any situation, especially when it comes to one's physical health.

The pain passed; then it returned worse than ever. I whispered to my wife, "I feel funny and think I need to get some fresh air." Rather than fall from my seat and startle the group, I quietly exited the rear door to the church. She quickly followed me outside because she had noticed me squirming in my seat and observed the strange look on my face. I took a few deep breaths. That seemed better... Then the pain hit me so hard again I was nearly driven to my knees. I caught myself on the tail gate of an F-150, or the ground would have caught me. By now my wife, Miranda, was getting more than a little concerned. She began to insist I go to the ER. But I simply was not ready, yet. Then like I had never had a pain at all, it was gone. But I couldn't quiet that small, still voice in the back of my mind saying, "Get to the hospital!"

The Rocky Ridge Quartet were singing at our church that night, and I really wanted to hear them, so I convinced Miranda to let me stay rather than head home early. I have ever been adept in the art of getting my way from a very early age. I also rationalized that there is no better place to die than at church. I have never feared dying because it is really not an end, but rather a beginning. They sang a song I'll never forget entitled "Kneel and Pray." We stayed for the entire song service, and did I suffer through it... physically speaking. I even pounded on my chest repeatedly to try and make the pain stop. I guess I was trying to knock whatever was hurting out of me, but this foolishness was to no avail. My doctors would later tell me I was lucky this didn't inadvertently cost me my life. Most aortic dissections are a result of blunt force trauma to the chest, such as impacting on a steering wheel in an accident. The pains continued to come and go. This is what made my situation so perplexing. One minute I felt as if an elephant were standing on my chest, and the next minute he stepped off. The problem was that he kept hopping back on me.

Fear will make one do things and act in ways one would not normally. For instance, if a dog is backed into a corner, he will bite you before a mean dog will because he is scared of no way out. My fear of what I might hear and be faced with at the hospital is what prevented me from going to the emergency room. Also adding to my dilemma was the physical state to which my body was rapidly deteriorating. However, even as death hovered around me, my physical appearance remained unchanged. Outwardly, I appeared to be the same old John. It still puzzles me how one can be so ill on the inside and never manifest a visible symptom. And even though I looked fine, something kept telling me, "Get to a hospital!"

Eureka! The effect of sin on the soul is a good analogy. It will rot a soul, yet no one other than God ever sees the harm it is doing which will ultimately end in death.

My wife and parents made a futile attempt to verbally force me to the emergency room that Sunday night. However, they were all thinking on their timetable, and a human being's clock will never coincide with God's stopwatch. His timing is always spot on and timed to the nanosecond. God was unfolding a lesson in Miraculous 101 which I will never forget. Given the time to process all I have been through, I now more clearly, but not fully, understand it. The old John would have reasoned, "Boy, that was another close call." Yet I could not dismiss this so easily because God wanted His hand upon my life fully realized this time around. The contemporary John began to view things in a different light. It was as if God told me: "Look, son, you almost got yourself killed with your hard head this time. I kept whispering to you to get to the hospital, but you thought you knew better than I. I only try to direct you because I love you. You disobeyed my clear direction for four days straight. These were not directions on getting to the beach; this was a matter of life and death. I allowed you to survive, against all odds, those four days so that you would have no doubt in your mind I had and continue to have My hand upon you. Without My provision you would not be here today, emergency surgery or not."

January 30. I carried rural route one in Brinson on Monday. As I cased the mail and got ready to serve my patrons, my pain returned. By this time I was getting as used to it as I could. It now felt like an old friend, the kind you let in the back door even though you want to pretend like you're not at home. I was getting a little winded, and my head started to hurt. So I ate four Advil and chugged a Coke, my usual prescription for whatever ailed me. But this time the old fix didn't work. Looking back, I now know why I was a Coke addict, the liquid kind. Some days I would only drink four or five, but most days it was a twelve pack or two three liter bottles. I needed the caffeine to get me through the day because my heart was unable to circulate my blood properly. Since my surgery I have not had even a swallow of Coke. That's not to say I haven't been tempted... I dragged myself around the route and finally came back to the Post Office. My Post Master even asked if I was feeling all right, to which I mumbled something about possibly pulling a muscle in my chest. Yeah, I pulled a muscle. Maybe I should get it checked out at the hospital, but I'll be fine.

February 1. I woke up Tuesday morning feeling like a champ. But try as I might, I simply could not shake the feeling that something was terribly wrong within me. Splitting wood always clears my head, so I ventured to the wood shed. I love the sound of an ax separating the wood grain in the crisp Fall air. I had a good pile of stove wood split when I nearly doubled over in agony. Out of the corner of my eye I saw my mother round the corner at the pump house, so I sucked it up again and began gathering the wood on bended knee.

"How are you feeling today?" she asked, the worry still evident in her tone. "I'm great!" I replied, lying through my teeth. She thought my wood gathering was a bit excessive, "Expecting it to freeze John?" "No ma'am, just want to be ready for the cold snap before Easter." After I neatly stacked the wood at our back door I spent the rest of the afternoon on the couch in a considerable level of pain. Lying there, I rationalized I must have really strained a muscle with all that wood work. That was a plausible explanation to my meddlesome mind. However, my mind was starting to wonder if that recurring voice telling me to "Get to the hospital" knew better than I what was best for me.

February 2. Wednesday my wife was off of work and she forced me no, constrained me, to go to my local physician. After a once over, he concluded I probably had pleurisy or, at worst, bacterial endocarditis. I breathed a little easier because both of these maladies are treatable with antibiotics. The doctor wrote me up some prescriptions, and I quickly tried to escape his observant eyes. The pain was hitting again, and I felt like it might bring tears to my eyes. He gripped my shoulder, looked me square in the eye, and pleaded with me to go to the hospital for more conclusive testing. Ugggh!!! There was that nasty little phrase again, and this time I wasn't simply hearing it in my head. As I tried to squirm past the doctor and into the hall, he told me of a gentleman who had suffered an aortic dissection. Unbeknown to us, this was exactly what I was presently experiencing.

I earned a Bachelor of Science in English and have read quite a few books in my lifetime. The foreshadowing by the doctor would later prove to be as ironic as a literary device in a well penned novel. As I stated earlier, fact is sometimes stranger than the best written fiction.

He then diagnosed my present condition and never knew it. "The guy's aorta dissected toward the inside, rather than toward the outside, or he would have died immediately." Died. Immediately. These two words echoed through the corridors of my mind. But still I continued to silence that little voice begging me to "Get to the hospital" as I hurried out the door of the doctors' office.

I now had heard it from a professional in the medical field that I probably had an illness which resulted in sharp, stabbing pains to the chest area. I neglected to mention to the doctor that it actually felt like I had an elephant standing on my chest, a tell-tell indicator of cardiac problems, rather than a knife sticking in it. The devil's always in the details. I proposed in my weak mind that from this point onward I was not going to complain of any more pain, no matter how bad it got. I would just grin and bear it. The biggest misconception I was solacing myself with was that the heart is on the left side of the chest. Remember in grade school when the teacher always said, "Put your right hand over your heart." To be accurate, we should place our hand in the center of our chest. After my recent crash course in anatomy I now know it really rests squarely behind the sternum. God, in His infinite wisdom, put it there to provide the most important organ in the body the maximum amount of protection possible. The body can live without many different components, like an arm, a gall bladder, an eye. Even if the brain is dead, your organs can still work together to support the body. But without a heart, there is no life. If I had paid better attention in safety and first aid at college, I would have probably retained this bit of important information regarding the location of said organ.

Back at home I started on my antibiotics and waited rather impatiently for them to start taking effect. As Wednesday evening prayer meeting approached, I simply didn't have the strength to go to church. I literally felt as if the life was draining out of my body. Miranda could see I still didn't feel well, so she stayed at home with me. The pain had never really left that afternoon, and it began to steadily increase. I held back the tears for as long as I could, but it was suddenly overwhelming. Nothing in my life had ever hurt that bad. I have a high threshold for pain; therefore she knew this was totally out of character for me. She even shed a few tears in a vain attempt to coax me out of my recliner and to the emergency room. I guess a good nick-name for me would be mule or jackass because I am definitely as stubborn as the animal. I pulled myself together enough to convince her I was all right. This was no easy task because by this time I was having trouble making myself believe I was all right. It was a performance worthy of academy award consideration. And that pesky little voice had taken on a stern tone when it implored me to "Get to the hospital before it is too late, son." Later that night, much later, I quietly cried myself to sleep.

February 3. Thursday morning I awoke to my wife brandishing a thermometer at me like a ringmaster with a whip in a lion's cage. It seems I had kept her awake all night with my groaning and tossing and turning. She would later tell me she had never seen me so restless or hot with fever. Everybody knows fevers rise in the evening and break in the morning. At eight A.M. my temperature was 104 degrees and showed no sign of stopping. I literally felt like my brain was that egg in the "this is your brain on drugs" add campaign from the 1980's. I could feel it starting to sizzle around the edges. She made me promise to call my mother, notify her of my worsened condition, get back to the doctor, and find a cure for this mystery illness I had seemingly contracted.

"Yeah, yeah, yeah," I muttered as I kissed her goodbye, and she reluctantly left for work. With her out the door I rolled over and tried to go back to sleep, thinking to myself, "I just need some bed rest and a big bowl of chicken noodle soup." Incidentally, why does it always have to be chicken noodle soup? Why couldn't it be tomato soup that is supposed to cure all ailments? Now I fully believe Satan and his minions had me in a snare with which they were planning to rob me of my life prematurely. And as I continued to disobey that little voice in my head, I was helping him. Still I kept hearing it repeat the same thing over and over, "Get to the hospital before it is too late!" While growing up, I was somewhat of a fatalist. One of my favorite sayings was, "Hell, I ain't gonna live to see 30 anyway." This almost became a self- fufilled prophecy.

Allow me to fast forward to the end and educate you about the ailment I was suffering. I would soon learn that my blood was not carrying oxygen to my brain as it should, thus severely diminishing my mental faculties. Four days had now passed since the initial onset of the pain in my chest. Although no one knows for sure, I will always believe that Sunday night at church was when I suffered the life-threatening dissection in my aorta. I knew nothing of this medical condition, especially not the signs and symptoms. I had never even heard of it, but I am a quick study.

Aortic dissections kill two out of 10,000 Americans each year, and they are most often seen in men ages 40-70. Eight out of ten patients die before they get treatment, and one of four die on the operating table. Left untreated, the likelihood of death within the first 48 hours is one percent per hour. Keep in mind I majored in English, not math; however, I have done my homework on these figures. I have calculated them long and hard, sometimes into the wee hours of the morning. If the dissection occurred on or around seven P.M. on Sunday, the odds I should have already been dead were hovering around 94 percent. For me, that seems pretty close to death. An untreated aortic dissection is not something an individual can simply get over or treat with antibiotics. The most notable case is John Ritter. Neither fame, fortune, nor faith can fix this silent killer once it passes the point of no return. If the dissection ever ruptures, you only have six beats of your heart to say goodbye. There are no exceptions. Even if the best, most proficient team of cardiovascular surgeons in the world already had the chest cavity cracked open and are ready to operate, if the dissection ruptures, they simply cannot work fast enough to stop the massive loss of blood. It is simply a matter of too much uncontrollable bleeding to overcome. Most survivors go to the emergency room at the initial onset of pain, but I was not so inclined.

The following statistics shocked me. Around 58.8 million Americans suffer from some form of heart disease. Every thirty-three seconds someone dies from a cardiovascular condition. An aortic dissection is defined as a condition in which there is bleeding into and along the wall of the aorta (the major artery from the heart). This condition may also involve abnormal widening or ballooning of the aorta, an aneurysm. The exact cause is unknown, but risks include atherosclerosis, hypertension, and traumatic injury, like blunt trauma to the chest as can be caused by hitting the steering wheel of a car during an accident.

Upon learning this, I have since wondered if the impact I took in the motorcycle accident had anything to do with the weakening of my aorta. It certainly could not have helped any. If I hadn't been in that accident, would I still have suffered the dissection? First it was disobedience to my earthly father, and then it was disobedience to the whisper of my Heavenly Father. In both cases, disobedience nearly cost me my life. These are things I have spent many restless nights contemplating.

One of my surgeons put in laymen's terms for me this explanation, "Picture a water hose. If it splits from the inside to the outside, all but the thin outer layer, you've got yourself a dissected water hose. However, if that outer layer ruptures, you've got a hose that won't hold pressure. Apply that elementary illustration to the aorta, and you get the picture. In the case of the hose, the well, pumping on an unlimited supply, will pump more water until someone turns the faucet off, but the heart operates with a finite amount of blood, eleven pints in the average human. It beats seventy times in a minute, forcing about 525 pounds of pressure through the aorta each hour. To put it mildly, a ruptured aorta is no good. The blood volume and rate of circulation will quickly be depleted. The life is in the blood, and without it we cannot live."

After I dragged myself out of bed that ominous Thursday morning, I proceeded to gather some wood to build a small fire to knock the chill out of the air. It was only three short steps from our hearth to the stack of wood kept inside our home during the winter. I squatted down to pick up the wood and turned around to head to the heater, I never knew what hit me. I was so affected by the lack of blood flow that I collapsed in the middle of my first step. I thought, "Boy! I must really have something nasty. I feel weak. I sure hope these antibiotics work. I don't want to have to go back to the doctor." By this point my head and the room had started to spin. Little did I know, I was about to have the doctor's visit of my life.

Enter my mother. It seems my wife had called her on the down-low, quite possibly saving my life. I am an only child; therefore I am extremely apt in the art of manipulation. She took one look at my present appearance, and I could see the fear in her eyes. The conversation was somewhat one-sided because I didn't get the chance to speak. Mom left me no room for argument as she announced, "John, pack an overnight bag. If this is pleurisy, you're too young to do irreparable damage to your lungs with your hard head. You're going to the hospital for some tests." No more pleading from that nice little voice in my head, finally a cooler head had prevailed. By this point we had all started to question if my mystery illness was in fact a lung infection. My pain was almost unbearable. I seriously needed some pain killers. I resigned myself to the fact that this was it; I would now have to face the dreaded hospital.

Eureka! My trip to the hospital is likened to some people's journey to salvation. I kicked against it until I had no strength left in me. This is exactly the point some stiff necked souls must come to before they can surrender to the fact that what they have been struggling against is Jesus Christ. He is the only one who can save them.

I still didn't want to go to the hospital, but I no longer had any strength to fight left in my body. Dad helped me into the car and basically flew me to my internal medicine specialist in Thomasville, Georgia. We were all now silently thinking the same thing. Whatever was wrong with me was far worse than we initially suspected. However, nobody was brave enough to verbalize the thought. Maybe what we didn't say wouldn't be true. Once at the doctor's office, I didn't have to wait long when the receptionist told Dr. Gee I was complaining of severe chest pain. Obviously from the look on my face the nurse could tell I was gravely ill. No pun intended. Dr. Gee rapidly ruled out several possible ailments and wasted no time in ordering an echocardiogram. An aortic dissection is a subtle medical anomaly that often goes undetected. It is routinely overlooked on standard evaluations and x-rays. There is no physical manifestation; therefore, even skilled doctors can miss this condition. God blessed me with a doctor who knew whatever I had, it was serious. He either acted on a hunch, or by simple deduction he knew I needed more thorough testing. Either way, he wasn't about to let me walk out of his office. I even tried to convince him I just needed some stronger antibiotics. I was no doubt a touch delirious. He didn't even nibble at my bait. This would prove to be a life-saving decision on his part.

In years past, I annually underwent an echocardiogram on my leaky bicuspid aortic valve to monitor my condition. This defect was never a problem for me, my mother, or my grandfather, but, I had neglected to have it checked in over eight years. In 1997 my cardiologist informed me of the growing expansion in my aorta. He told me I would probably need to consider surgery in the coming years. This thought paralyzed me with fear. I still remember the way my mom reacted when we discovered I had a heart defect. Yet my parents always tried to reassure me, or maybe it was for their reassurance, that it was a minor problem. Their initial reaction to that discovery led me to believe something serious would eventually come of my "minor" problem. Open heart surgery had always been my worst fear in life. I often thought, "God just let me die before I have to be split open." So when the doctor simply suggested

I may need to consider surgery, I decided then that I would never go back to him. And I did not. So long it had been since I had seen him that when Dr. Gee's office tried to contact him for my records they were informed that he had long since retired. If you are thinking my parents are to blame, they are not. They were persistent over those eight years in their attempts to get me to go for checkups. However, I was now an adult. My dad told me when I turned eighteen that he was taking his hands off me. He said "John, you are an adult now. If you make a mistake, you are going to be responsible for it." My neglected regular checkups were definitely one mistake I made as an adult. The present echo revealed that over the years when I neglected to check my valve, it had been doing some growing, quite a bit. It had expanded from a normal measurement of 2.6cm to the abnormal size of 7.9cm. This was not great news, but it was not a death sentence either. That condition would have still been considered an elective surgery. This expansion is what led to my Coke habit. It was robbing me of my energy and stamina. However, the deeply disturbing factor discovered during the echo was the deadly dissection in the wall of my aorta.

Dr. Gee's nurse took me next door in a wheelchair to undergo the echocardiogram. As I tried to lie still and relax for the technician, my chest pain reached a level which I thought was literally going to kill me. Have you ever been in so much pain you thought you would die? Now there was no respite from the pain. The elephant was no longer stepping on and off; he had started doing jumping jacks. With each beat of my heart, the pain was intensifying. I couldn't stand it any longer; I began to weep uncontrollably as a result of my bodily anguish. The technician solemnly questioned me, "Are you sure your doctor knows you are having chest pain this severe?" By this point I was not sure what I knew and did not know. My mom and dad were both in the room with me, because I had been reduced to a scared little boy about to get his first shot. At this moment we all simultaneously knew my pain was a result of something taking place which was terribly wrong.

In the middle of that revelation in walked my new cardiologist, Dr. Karas. Even though he had never seen me, he had already heard of me through my mother, who had been under his care for several years. During all my previous echocardiograms, the technicians taking the pictures and video always commented on the changes to my defect as they took the pictures. Heretofore, it was always, "Everything looks good. Nothing has drastically changed. Did you have eggs for breakfast?" It was always a lighthearted mood. When I nervously asked my new acquaintance, "How does everything look buddy?" he evasively said, "I can't tell yet. We'll have to wait for your doctor to have a look see." He was too tight lipped, and his voice betrayed him. I knew in my heart I was about to face my worst fear in life.

Dr. Karas had been on rounds at Archibald Memorial Hospital, directly across the street from my present location. As I lay squirming on the examination table, he hurried into the room. I realized whatever the technician discovered on the echo definitely got his undivided attention. Before the echocardiogram I had extensive blood work done in the lab. As I alluded to earlier, this speedy analysis revealed my blood was not properly delivering oxygen to my brain or the rest of my vital organs. This explained why I collapsed at home and why I literally did not have the brainpower to recognize how sick I really was.

When Dr. Karas came in, he never even looked at the results of the echocardiogram. Thus, the technician had to have seen what was happening in my aorta, and I surmised he briefed the doctor over the phone when he had momentarily stepped out the door. Dr. Karas broke the unsettling news as gently as he could. "John, nice to meet you, Mr. and Mrs. Roberts; I've got bad news and good news. First, your aorta has severely dissected. Second, this requires an immediate surgical procedure to save your life. We must act quickly. Don't worry. I'm going to get you to the right people and get you all fixed up. It's lunch time in Tallahassee, so I'm going to have to make some calls to get a team ready for your arrival. You'll immediately go into surgery upon your arrival. Don't worry, I know some great people down there. They will do all they can to save your life." I asked one question, "Are you sure I have to have surgery?" "Yes, John, you must."

With those words he excused himself and disappeared in a blur of his long white coat, leaving my parents and myself to break down in silent solitude. Yet it never happened to me. In shock and total disbelief, I heard my mother start to softly sob across the room. Something had hurt her little boy that she simply could not kiss and make better. My father momentarily lost his composure because he understood exactly the ramifications of a dissected aorta. He has read <u>Grey's Anatomy</u> enough times to possess a self-awarded medical degree. During my formative years I never fully understood why anyone would subject himself to such punishment. After I grew into a man, I understood.

My mom and dad came from poor families. Growing up in the 1940's, one was either among the "haves" or the "have nots." My forefathers were with the "nots." My grandparents had everything they could ever hope for in the Lord, but they had little when it came to the worldly standard. Adrian Rogers defined wealth as anything money can't buy and death can't take away. By this definition my lineage was extremely wealthy. You can't buy the kind of love they passed down from generation to generation, and death can't end the bond love like that creates. As a direct result of their meager childhoods, my parents sacrificed their wants and desires to afford me the best life possible.

They put their dreams on hold so that they could prepare a secure future for their child. However, in my estimation they never really forgot about those early childhood desires. They were simply moved to the back burner. Dad has told me how he used to watch the big planes fly over our small family farm and dream of being the pilot behind the yoke. He would sit all afternoon and ponder who was at the controls and where they were going. After he secured a stable job, he took flight lessons and learned how to fly. After a lot of hard work and patience, he was finally able to buy himself a small Cessna. His dream came true. It became clear to me he could have also been a doctor if he had been financially able to attend medical school. Being an avid reader my entire life, I discovered dad liked to dig deep the first time I ever opened his copy of Grey's Anatomy. In my teenage years, I knew he missed his calling when he continued to buy the new editions of the famed medical journal each time it was reprinted. "Why would anyone who is not a doctor sit around and read this stuff for kicks?" I often asked myself. I formed a logical answer in my mind. Why did I read Hemingway and Fitzgerald; simply because I enjoyed them. And the same principle applied to my dad; he simply enjoyed learning about the human body in the same way I enjoyed two of my favorite authors. My mother has never really discussed her early ambitions, but from what I have gathered from my father, I think she would have liked a career in the nursing field. She even remarked on occasion during my collegiate years that she ought to just go back to school with me. I thought she was just having a hard time letting go of me.

Life is what happens while we are planning for the future. One minute we graduate, the next we are married, and then it is all about providing for our family. Once that family has an addition of a newborn, our dreams and desires are no longer important. The top priority becomes that little baby with which we have been blessed. This is what happened in the case of my parents. But life always seems to come full circle in my opinion. In a way they both ended in the medical field. It does not require a doctorate in English to take great pleasure in reading and writing. And so it is with other fields of interest. My parents are volunteers with Hospice, a wonderful organization that helps terminally ill patients and their families. They are also caregivers to elderly people. These people are too old to safely live alone, and their families do not want to place them in a nursing home. What are doctors and nurses when all is said and done? They are caregivers. However, I digress...

As the gravity of the diagnosis settled in, I was the one who remained calm in the eye of the storm. I suppose one reason was because I was the one who the unfortunate situation was swirling around. Even though hurricanes are destructive and violent, their eye is calm and smooth. I was the one whose emotions always got out of hand. In the face of death, it still amazes me how collected I remained. How did I manage to remain together? I never did. God did it all for me through Jesus Christ and the indwelling Holy Spirit. When my earthly father couldn't comfort himself, let alone me, my Heavenly Father spoke directly to my soul. This is the only time in my life I can actually say I heard God speak to me. He softly, yet strongly, whispered II Corinthians 12:9 to me in His own words that fit my exact need at that moment in time. I heard His voice just as if He had been standing on Earth right beside me. It was the sweetest voice I have ever heard. God said, "John, my grace is sufficient for thee: for my strength will be made perfect in your weakness. Most gladly therefore should you rather glory in your infirmities, that the power of Christ may rest upon you. Don't worry my son, you're in good hands. Everything is going to be ok." From that second until I shook off my anesthesia, I felt no fear, no doubt, no anxiety, and no worry. I was surrounded by nothing but the mercy, grace, strength, and love of God. I did not have a mystical vision. An angel did not speak to me. The clouds did not roll back like a scroll. Yet I knew I was safely and securely in my Savior's hand. And He in turn was and always is in His Father's hand from which a believer cannot be pulled by any shape, form, or fashion. My deep faith in the hand of God upon my life from an early age is what anchored my unshakable confidence. If I had never been born again, I would not have experienced that assurance.

My soul cried out at the most desperate time in my life. I was so distraught that I couldn't even think of words to pray. When Dr. Karas diagnosed my condition, my mind reeled, considering the possible scenarios that might be the outcome. I remember not even being able to pray a single word to God. Then an important promise came to mind from Romans 8:26, "the Spirit also helps our infirmities: for we know not what we should pray for as we ought: but the Spirit itself maketh intercession for us with groaning which cannot be uttered." In my darkest hour when I did not know if I would live through my next heartbeat, the Holy Spirit in me was speaking for me to Christ who was in turn pleading my cause to our heavenly Father. Christ has never moved from His seat at the right hand of God, and He makes intercessions on our behalf. Theoretically peace is a wonderful idea. However, attaining or achieving it on your own is not practical. Of oneself will always come and go, but given of God it will endure anything. This peace, which only God grants, is how I knew everything was going to be all right. As a child of the King, one need never worry about anything whether it is in life or death.

Dr. Karas reentered to announce my departure for the trauma unit. Once there, I was given a shot of morphine for my pain. The drug never did dull my mental alertness because I was far too alert from adrenaline, but it did finally stop my severe chest pain. This was a welcome relief because I had been assaulted by this pain for four days. I begged for a nice lift to Tallahassee aboard a life-flight helicopter, which would have been sweet to recount here; however, I was headed down on an ambulance. My dad was intent on accompanying me in the ambulance, but the doctors would not budge. I quickly reminded him he needed to get mom to Tallahassee because she was in no shape to drive. We quickly said farewell, and I was on my way.

On that ride to Tallahassee, I regained my composure, and I was able to speak openly and honestly with God.

Eureka! This is what God always desires of His children. He doesn't want lip service and rote memorization but rather what is in our heart. He already knows what is in there anyway. How pleased He must be when we are honest with Him and ourselves.

"Lord, you know I'm only 28 years old. I've got a young wife, a mother, father, grannie, mema, and granddaddy, as well as a host of family and friends. I'm not ready to leave them, but you know better than I what is best for me. I know you hold my temporal and eternal future in your hand. See me through this if it be in your will for me to live. However, if my number is up, I'll gladly leave it all behind. Please give Miranda and my family the peace and strength you are imparting to me just now. Whatever the outcome, please continue to surround them with your love. As Job said in the middle of his tribulation, "Though you slay me, yet will I trust you"" (Job 13:15).

Thanking God for His many blessings is a prayer that comes effortlessly. But the aforementioned petition was mentally, physically, and spiritually draining. I was more in touch with God than I had ever been in my life, and at the same time I was quickly approaching death. With every beat of my heart I literally felt the lifeblood dying within me. My heart was ready to give up, but my spirit told it to have faith. I meant that prayer with all my heart, soul, and strength. I do not know how all the prayer warriors who stood in the gap for me during this same time appealed to God, but I think it must have been in the same vein. No pun intended. Just thinking hypothetically about one's death is emotionally draining and disturbing; however, when the genuine possibility of one's impending demise sets in, the weight of the situation is almost overwhelming. Yet moment by moment God sustained me with comfort from

His Holy Word. I had read it all my life, but never had I needed to apply it to such a critical personal circumstance. However, I was quickly beginning to fathom God's promises and His Holy Word in ways I never even imagined. Just as a wave of sorrow and self-pity was about to break on me to drag me down to the bottom, there was my mighty God with His wings of protection spread wide to shelter me form the noisome pestilence with His living word. Brother Paul faced hard times. His words in II Corinthians 12:10 brought me more hope, strength, and comfort. He wrote, "Therefore I take pleasure in infirmities, in reproaches, in necessities, in persecutions, in distresses for Christ's sake: for when I am weak, then am I strong."

Eureka! When I am weak, then am I strong. Being a sickly child, I had quoted this my entire life, but I'd never truly been weak like now. One must embrace one's weakness and fully surrender thoughts of overcoming anything alone to experience the strength of God.

Finances, cars, homes, material possessions, worldly accolades, or future plans never entered my mind as I was knocking on Heaven's door. It was thoughts of my relationship with Jesus Christ and my family. That's it, end of story. Everything else just faded away. It is really sad that it took a brush so close with death to make me fully realize and comprehend this important truth. Christ does not just want to be number one at the end of our earthly lives when we are out of time to serve Him. He wants to be number one every second, minute, and hour of each day while we can be a light pointing others to the knowledge and saving grace He provides through His redemptive work on the cross.

As the paramedics quickly wheeled me, my wife jogging alongside, into Cardiovascular Surgical Intensive Care Unit room number 1177, she knew this was not routine for more testing. My parents were a little less than truthful with her to ensure her safe arrival at the hospital. They had her boss tell her I wanted her to be there with me as I underwent more tests. Some tests. The ambulance I was traveling on, at 90-100 mph, did not arrive before her. I know her Mustang GT must have been galloping because both vehicles traveled approximately the same distance. The only difference was she got lost on a one way street, had lunch time traffic to navigate, and no flashing lights or sirens. Somehow she still beat me to the hospital by a good fifteen minutes. During that time the nurses' desk must have thought they had a lunatic on their hands. The medical community has become silent when speaking with anyone regarding a patient over the past few years. I understand the need for privacy, but this was not one of the times it was called for. Miranda was trying to locate and get some information on one Robert John Roberts, her husband no less, and all the desk could tell her was that they had an Ezra Roberts in route from Thomasville, Georgia. She was truly unnerved when I saw her. I just wanted to know how she got to the hospital before me. "How fast were you driving honey? Because we were doing like a buck twenty!" She never told me her speed and still says she can't remember how fast she was going. I think she worries the truth could give me a heart attack.

I explained as best I could, with my then limited knowledge of the condition, what was really going on; the punch line was I was having heart surgery immediately. Her eyes welled up with tears as the nurses began starting intravenous lines, hooking up various monitors, and generally making a pin cushion of my body. Then I could see her determine to be strong for me. She fought back the tears, regained her composure, and asked with her loving eyes, "What can I do?" She didn't even have to verbalize her thoughts; I knew what she was thinking. I assured her, "I'm going to be ok. God will shelter us through this storm. He's already promised me that this morning. I can't explain it, but I know in my heart everything is gonna work out for the best." We only had a few minutes together as she helped me out of my clothes and into my stylish hospital gown before my head surgeon, Dr. Saint, entered the room. He definitely has the right surname because in my eyes he will always be a saint to me. In those few moments our life together flashed before my eyes, and I didn't have a single regret. The only mystery in my mind was why the highlight reel didn't last longer.

Upon Dr. Saint's arrival, the day took on a critical feel. No pun intended. A nurse hurried my arriving parents into the room. They were not on a GT; they were on Big Bertha. Dr. Saint spoke calmly, but quickly. He spoke to them, more than me, as I was pretty looped by this point. "The surgery John is about to undergo is one I do on occasion." I thought,

"Great! Leave it to me to arrive on the day he wants to do his next occasional operation."

Then he spouted the statistics of the situation "His problem can be repaired, but we must operate now. As soon as I finish here, I'm going to scrub up and my team is going to work to save his life. He has a 50 percent mortality rate and a 50 percent chance this surgery could end his life." I'm thinking, "Quit referring to me in the third person! I'm laying right here, and I can hear everything you are saying about me!"

Dr. Saint also went over the possible complications, "He could be left in a vegetative state, suffer a stroke, experience organ failure, get irreversible amnesia, possible brain damage, suffer a heart attack, have various degrees of paralysis, be completely paralyzed, or even die on the operating table. But don't worry. We are going to do everything in our power to fix his problem. I'll treat him like he was my own son." I couldn't take it anymore. I had to speak up, "Don't worry about the possible brain damage, Doc. I already covered that one a few years back." To which no one even smiled for me. At least I thought it was funny...

I speculated to myself, "This is gonna be like the pill you have to take to live that could possibly give you diarrhea, fatigue, sweaty palms, constipation, dry mouth, water retention, ankle swelling, headaches, vomiting, abdominal cramping, mood swings, hair growth in unwanted places, and lots of other side effects we don't have time to mention." Suffice to say, I came away from the surgery with a host of quirks I didn't expect, but as dad says, "That's the price you pay for pepperoni." Above all, I did come away from it with my life.

Back to room 1177, "Mr. Roberts, please sign on the dotted line." In other words, if you die, we're not going to be liable. I half joking, half hoping, asked Dr. Saint if he was sure another round of antibiotics wouldn't clear this thing up. He seemed humorless and still didn't crack a smile. So I signed, not because I wanted to but because I was facing a certain death sentence.

Eureka! Being born again is like unto my operation. It is something many people do not want to experience, but without it they are facing a death sentence. However, Christ has paid the fine we could not pay. It is up to us to accept His gift. We are beings with the privilege of choice. If I had refused the surgery, I would have surely died. If you fail to accept Christ, you will face a fate far worse than death here on Earth.

As I lay dying with Dr. Saint and his skilled team gathered around him, I knew I was where God had placed me and wanted me to be for this operation. I thought, "With a Saint in the operation room how can I be going wrong?" No pun intended. By this point I had certainly been affected by the shock of the morning, and no doubt the drugs were starting to take their toll as I headed to the Land of Nod. I don't know if anyone else noticed, but to me the surgical team seemed to appear angelic in a sense. It could have been my mind playing tricks on me. It could have been the drugs. Or I could have possibly seen the wings of angels hovering behind them. Even the doctors later told me I came as close to death without actually dying as anyone wants to get. I have no doubts they were angels all around me to protect me that day. Regardless, I envisioned bright white wings as they hovered over me, anxious to begin the task that lay ahead. "Please say your goodbyes for now. Don't worry son; you're in good hands. Everything's going to be ok."

It occurred to me, "Wow. That's exactly what God said."

I thought I had just heard the most enormous run-on sentence of my life, and I can make a pretty big run-on myself. Did he even take a breath during all those words? Dr. Saint's words hit me on a guttural level. Yet my emotions still did not overwhelm me. I was a stone-faced stoic, in shock still, or in complete denial of what was happening to me. To the contrary, it was none of the above. I was in the caring, capable, compassionate hands of my Creator. I had to be strong for my wife and parents. They had enough to lament without worrying about comforting me. God keeps His promises to His children, and that was all I needed to console me. My emotions didn't need to add to my family's panic. Death was never really an option in my mind, but if it happened on the operating table, I didn't want them to look back on my last moments on Earth and see me in fear. I wanted them to see a fighter who fought a good fight but whose time was simply cut short. They would come to understand that God must have had a greater purpose for me to accomplish in death rather than in life. To live is Christ, but to die is gain. God's matchless grace continued to sustain me. It was the only way I was able to survive.

Now we were in the short rows as my dad always says. The clock was ticking, and it was ticking fast. No pause button, and there was no more slow motion. It was full steam ahead toward the end of a track to which no one but God could see the depot at the end. The nurses came and briskly rolled me to the holding room to await surgery. "Ok folks, this is as far as you can accompany him. Say your goodbyes", they announced to my wife and parents. This was really it, I was about to undergo a surgery I might not survive. I refused to say goodbye. I simply stated, "I will see you all on the other side or say hello to Heaven." The fear began to choke the life out of me, and instantly it was gone.

People say, "Ah, angels... there's no such thing as angels." But I believe differently. I know my guardian angel and a special spiritual tactical team waged war to protect my physically racked and dying body on February 3, 2005. As soon as Satan attempted to gain a foothold or cast a fiery dart at me, the advance was squashed by my invisible protectors. Looking back, I can see my guardian angels, in my mind's eye, surrounding me. They are standing in a tight 360 degree formation, shoulder to shoulder, with their backs toward me. They positioned themselves so closely not even Satan himself could squeeze through to harm one hair on my head. That is the angelic hedge of protection the Bible promises, not some hocus-pocus-mumbo-jumbo but a real spiritual wall no evil force can penetrate.

It starts to get a little blurry for me here, so stay with me. Miranda, Mom, and Dad were in the room alone with me now. I asked for someone to please pray over me. Billy Graham could not have comforted me more with one of his prayers. Daddy, my mentor in the Christian faith prayed, they all prayed, just like I was praying. God's throne was being bombarded with prayers already from one little phone call my Dad made to his baby brother.

I'll never forget that call from the trauma unit in Thomasville before I was loaded onto the ambulance. "Scott," Dad said fighting back the emotion in his voice and his tears, "John's got a little problem. It's his heart. It's fixable, but it's serious. We need you to pray, like never before. Make some calls and get a hold of as many people as you can. Can you do that for me?" Only God truly knows the number of prayers that went up on my behalf from that one call, not prayers that stop at the ceiling but prayers that screamed upward like supersonic rockets directly to the throne of God. I know God heard them and answered them. Were it not for those prayers, I would not be here today.

Eureka! When someone is on trial, the judge always seems to be more lenient when the accused has supporters there for him. Their witness can even influence the judge's sentencing. I was being tried by fire, as the Bible says. God was and is the judge. Satan was the district attorney seeking to have me put to death. Those who were pleading my case to

The Judge were my defense team. They no doubt made a favorable impression.

Kisses were forthcoming, and then I was left all alone in that cold sterile room. I mused that they must have put me in the cafeteria freezer. My wife and parents were escorted to the waiting room where they held vigil from 4:30 until shortly after midnight when Dr. Saint came out to tell them of my successful operation. They did get updates via telephone from a nurse in the operating room. I wouldn't have traded places with any of them. I don't want to even imagine what they must have gone through each time the phone rang. Having to wonder, if I were dead, why it was taking so long, were they through, and what was going on back there? It must have been rough. I packed out the waiting room with my friends and family. At least I know I can draw a crowd.

After my anesthesiologist told me it was "lights out," I do not remember anything, not even counting backwards from ten. I have no memories at all until I got out of the cardiovascular surgical intensive care unit. I later learned they gave me the drug Versed, something the nurses refer to as "milk of amnesia." Believe me that it works just like it sounds it would. The first days in the private room are a blur at best. I was told a lot of what went on by my wonderful wife and other eyewitness accounts. Therefore, as I have no memory of these things, the next few paragraphs will come from memories shared with me from those who watched over me. I do recall a few moments in the fog. I remember being surrounded by nothing but love, more love than I have ever felt in my entire life. Also the mood was always light, never dark or depressing. I guess if my situation unnerved somebody, it was understood they needed to get out of the room for my sake. Nobody wanted me to be under any stress during this trying time of my recovery. Ah yes, it was the best of times; it was the worst of times. My family, friends, and medical staff truly rose to the occasion during a most difficult time in my life.

February 4, 2005. The nurses said I would probably be unconscious for at least a full day before I ever showed any signs of regaining conscious, let alone speaking to anybody. However, they met me at a weak moment no doubt. I regained consciousness the morning after the surgery, bright eyed and bushy tailed, just like I had been asleep at home in my own bed. My attending nurse began to ask me questions. "Mr. Roberts, do you know any of these people?" "Of course I do, those are my peeps," I tried to say, but the breathing tube would not allow me to speak clearly so it all sounded like the teacher on Charlie Brown. "Wonk wonk. Wonk wonk wonk." "Are you in any pain?" "No elephants in this room, lady. Just lots of pretty colors." More Charlie Brown. I quickly motioned for a pen and paper with which to communicate. I had just nearly died, and I was ready to say something monumental. However, I didn't get to use it because they said if I was that alert it was time to come off the respirator. They want patients breathing on their on as soon as possible. My family told me my first words were, "Are you ready for a baby?" That's still hard for me to believe...

So far so good; however, I was still a long way from being back to my old self. That is one thing I had such a hard time with during my slow recovery. People do not just bounce back into the daily grind after they have their chest cracked open. Heart patient should never really return to the way they were living. Chances are they were doing something that was not conducive to their good health in the first place such as smoking, drinking excessively, not eating right, or abusing their body with a bad diet. They must come to the realization that they are not the same people they were before heart surgery. I now live a better life than I did before, but I have had to make adjustments.

Normally after my particular operation blood and fluid accumulate in the chest cavity. This requires the chest being reopened to suction the fluids out to prevent infection. I had two drainage tubes running out of my torso to allow the excess fluids to escape from my body. Sometimes they work properly, and sometimes they simply get clogged. There was a lot of waiting, watching, and praying on the part of my family. The more the chest is reopened, the longer it takes to recover. Miraculously, my fluid build up was minimal, and my chest never had to be opened a second or third time. This was yet another miracle inside the miracle that God had already performed in my situation. My great nurses, Stacey in particular, kept a watchful eye on my drainage levels to ensure they remained within their acceptable parameters.

Getting paid to do a job is only fair, but to go above and beyond the call of duty is a quality that is sorely lacking in our modern day society. Most people simply want to show up for work, do as little as possible, and take home a pay check at the end of the week. If we all did our jobs as if they were unto the Lord, our workforce would be much more efficient, not to mention productive. As I began to recover, I shared many conversations with my nurses. Working in an intensive care unit must stimulate one's faith as miracles happen here routinely for all to see. I discovered many of them were Christians simply by asking them. How hard is that? It requires very little time or effort on our part, but so many times we fail to witness to others who may be lost and headed to Hell. Where would I be if those people who witnessed to me had been too busy to do so? It scares me to even think about it.

My selfless concern for my family is the number one quality the nurses noticed in me. During my time in CVSICU, cardiovascular surgical intensive care unit, I do not remember anything I said, but the staff all remarked that I was more preoccupied with my wife's wellbeing than I was my own. Each time she would excuse herself to go to the restroom, they told me I kept telling them how bad I felt that she had to go through this. If I were simply assuming to be concerned, I could have been mistaken. However, it was not my imagination because other people took note of my actions. This is a change for the better I still work on daily. A life for self is really no life at all.

Eureka! This is the true definition of joy.

Jesus
Others
Yourself

Yet Webster defines it as "intense happiness or great delight." God's dictionary will always differ from that of a man. Happiness is circumstantial. It will always come and go, but joy is the product of a life that pleases God. True joy is a fruit of the Spirit which no situation can take away.

The premise of this work was to declare the goodness of God and share my struggles with others so that they would know they were not the only ones to experience hard times. I put pen to paper in this undertaking because I communicate much better through the written word than I do verbally. When I write, I have the luxury of shaping and honing my words. When I am talking one on one with someone, I usually think of what I should have said a week later. And now, a byproduct of deep sedation for the surgery, I often lose my train of thought during daily conversation. It is extremely frustrating to have a point to make, but only to have it vanish from my mind completely. Witnessing was important in the years before my surgery, but I just didn't feel comfortable invading a strangers' life on a spiritual level. That meant getting out of my comfort zone. I felt one needed to get to know people before sharing the plan of Salvation with them. I now understand it is our greatest mission in life to step out of our comfort zone every time the opportunity presents itself.

We only have a limited number of years, months, weeks, days, hours, and seconds on this Earth from our birth. This is why it is imperative to always be aware of opportunities to work in our Father's kingdom. One day, and sooner than we think, our privilege to labor in the harvest will be over, and the sun will set on our life here on Earth. In Luke 10:2, Christ tells us "The harvest truly is great, but the labourers are few: pray ye therefore the Lord of the harvest, that he would send forth labourers into his harvest." My problem is that I often pray to the Lord about a situation without ever putting my feet to my petition. It should be our number one priority in life to toil in the approaching harvest. Yet far too often Satan blinds us with the business of busyness in this world. It is not difficult for him becausee he can appear as an "angel of light" (II Corinthians 11:14). We work hard to provide a future for our family. We run here and there, taking the kids to every extracurricular activity known to man. And at the end of the day, have we really been busy seeking God's will, or has Satan distracted us only to thwart God's plan for one more day?

My loving wife read scriptures to me during my stay in CVSICU. She could have read a comic book; I would have never known the difference. However, in Isaiah 55:11, God promises, "So shall my word be that goeth forth out of my mouth: it shall not return to me void, but it shall accomplish that which I please, and it shall prosper in the thing whereto I sent it." God knew I needed His word replanted in my fertile mind for the troublesome days that lay ahead of me.

I received a book titled Anchors of Hope by Sandi Banks. Several times after I came home I attempted to read this short book, but I could never get into it. The time wasn't right yet. Then one day as I was having a pity party deep in the doldrums of depression, I picked it up and read it in one afternoon. It did wonders for my melancholy state of mind. I strongly recommend it for anyone facing a struggle or hard time. Other than the Bible, this was the most helpful book I could find after my surgery. That is another reason I penned this memoir. I searched high and low and was never able to find a book that addressed life after heart surgery. Even though I cannot remember Miranda's words, I now know they were vital to my mental health. After she went back to work, at home alone with my reflections most of the day, I faced some tough thoughts. Six weeks after my operation, as I sat contemplating suicide day after day, I finally had to ask for help. Without the help I received, I probably wouldn't be here today.

My doctors warned me that I would face depression in the days ahead after I left the hospital. Post traumatic stress has been found to be experienced by more than 15 percent of heart-attack survivors. This disorder slows recovery and increases the chance of a second attack. I didn't have a heart-attack; I had something far worse according to my doctors. I should not have been so quick to dismiss their warning. No longer was I happy to be alive; I just thought I should be dead, and the sooner the better. My depression was draining the desire to live right out of me. I never breathed a word of my mental state to my family; I feared they would be so disappointed in me. At my last visit to my surgeon, as I was about to walk out the door, it hit me. I thought, "John, you know something is deeply wrong. Don't repeat the same mistake you made with your heart problem. Tell him how you really feel." I stopped in the doorway, turned around, and told Dr. Bixler I was seriously contemplating suicide. We had a long in depth talk. I had no intention of going through with suicide, but I had no control over the thought repeatedly entering my mind. I was scared that the desire would overpower my will.

Dr. Bixler explained what was occurring in my confused mind. He told me my body had literally gone through hell. I also learned the body can go on forever without sleep, but at some point the mind must shut down, or it will pay the price of sleep deprivation. I erroneously thought with my mended heart that I was running on an endless supply of energy, which was not true. The intensive care unit is like perpetual day. The patients are sedated so there is no need to turn off the lights to sleep. This also helps the nurses easily see everything they need to see in a critical environment. A nurse administers a shot to induce a peaceful night's sleep. This nonexistent night had my sleep cycle totally out of rhythm. My body knew it needed rest, but my mind told my body the exact opposite. I was staying up all hours of the night and hardly napping any during the day after I returned home. Soon sleep deprivation had turned me into a ball of rage and angst. I was angry at the world, and the bad part was I didn't even know why.

This sounds like a lot of young adults I know today. Lack of sleep will affect anybody even though one may not be aware of the change that is taking place. Behavioral patterns are affected when the body does not get the proper rest it needs. The neurons which control the brain begin to misfire when they are not given adequate time to regenerate.

Some organs have the ability to regenerate even when a person is not sleeping as long as those organs are not in use, for example with a broken leg. This process could be accomplished while lying awake, in a relaxed atmosphere. Thinking functions may not seem necessary in a relaxed state, but the brain is not capable of resting and recharging while it is still "turned on." The brain must be completely "switched off" from the realm of consciousness to get the proper recharging it needs. In short, we must sleep to ensure our proper mental health. This is a reason methamphetamine addicts commit unimaginable acts after a week long meth binge. The effects of the drug are only amplified by the loss of sleep.

It was not the stranger on the street who had to deal with my bad attitude but rather my wife who was waiting on me hand and foot. Looking back, I think I lashed out at her because she was doing all the things for me I used to be able to do for myself. It is not easy to transition from independence to dependence. For six long weeks I couldn't lift anything heavier than a gallon of milk. That's frustrating. She bore the brunt of my mental meltdowns when she got home from a hard day's work. They say you hurt those you are closest to, and this is exactly what happened in my case. I spoke with family members of others who had undergone heart surgery, and they echoed these same sentiments. It may be hard to understand how I could bite the hand that was literally feeding me, but that is what was happening. When Miranda would cook supper, it wasn't what I wanted. Or if I cooked a little something, she may not be hungry. Rather than take it at face value, a lack of appetite, I took it as a personal insult to the meal I had prepared. This was totally out of character for me. In times past, I was just glad she took the time to cook something for me, regardless of the dish. If she was not hungry, I simply ate without her. When she did the chores I normally did, she never did them the way I would have done them. My boxers weren't folded right or my shirts were not facing the right way in my closet. The problems I began creating were quickly becoming absurd. Thankfully, this only lasted for a few days before I got professional help from my doctor.

Men are often afraid of things, but they usually never admit their fear. I am not sure if it is pride, anxiety of the unknown, or what it is that specifically prevents us from seeking help in difficult situations. It's probably a combination of all of the above coupled with the society we grow up in. I've always heard older men making the comment, "Man up. You've got to toughen up if you ever want to be a man." They always imply that you must face things on your own, or it makes you less of a man. However, I know men are afraid to ask for help, of any sort, even when they know they need it. I did not stutter. I said it, and I consider myself a man's man. Any man who has had his sternum sawed in half with a stainless steel saw can call himself a man's man. In my humble opinion it takes a real man to face what he fears, disclose them to someone who understands the problem, and get the help he needs to overcome the situation.

A heart surgeon who has seen numerous cases other than mine told my wife and father how brave I was to speak up about my mental state. I majored in English, minored in sociology, and humanities; therefore, I learned much in regard to the human experience during my collegiate years. Being a Christian and student of the Bible since the age of five has also educated me deeply about human existence. I realized that if the mind is sick, the body it controls will suffer. Men must get over this machismo mentality and learn to ask for help when it is needed, or we run the highly probable risk of creating a dilemma we cannot handle or solve alone.

I experienced and realized this truth firsthand. This is not a hypothesis I read in a medical journal. It is a fact I learned in the school of hard knocks called life. When God has just delivered you from the jaws of death through a life threatening surgery as he did me, there is nothing Satan would like more than for you to end your life prematurely. Then he could throw God's mercy up in His face. He could argue, "See, God, I told you he wouldn't appreciate your kindness. Just look at how he has repaid you. You should have let me take his life before when I tried to." I have talked with patients in my situation who told me they turned to the wrong places for peace and answers, answers to questions they didn't even know how to ask. I hope that is as clear as mud. If you have never gone through a heart surgery, it will be hard for you to relate to what I am saying.

There are a lot of emotions and questions that go through the mind one never really understands. According to doctors anytime the heart is disturbed it wreaks havoc on all aspects of the human body, especially the mind. All the senses and mental faculties experience a turmoil that is hard to explain. Alcohol, drugs, or any number of other various self-destructive measures will not help one cope with matters a brain cannot comprehend. Most of these vices are just slow capitulation, long term suicide. God has burdened me to share the truth of what I experienced. The truth is that Satan attacked me mentally with the implicit thought of suicide.

I dabbled in a lot of things I shouldn't have in my younger days. Suffice to say, the pleasure of sin for a season enticed me to do things I knew were wrong. I experimented with the common vices and even some that were not so common. Thankfully, I realized that sin always brings forth fruit, and its fruit is death. If I had not seen the futility down those avenues early on, I would have taken a ride on that street car named desire at some point later in life. The desire of the heart will manifest itself at some point in time. One cannot ignore the burning inside but for so long. There is only one way not to worry about sin controlling one's life. It must not be allowed to fester like a cancer in the soul.

Eureka! An ounce of prevention is worth a pound of cure. This was the case with my heart trouble, in both situations. We need regular physical checkups to ensure our good health. But daily spiritual examinations are far more necessary to prevent long term ramifications in our lives.

We must confess our sins daily and properly see them for what they really are, rebellion against God. If not, they will affect our relationship with God. I will not catalog my sins here; I make my confessions directly to God. I am a Baptist. God gets no glory when we focus on our tawdry past. Suffice to say I have received my fair share of forgiveness because I struggled with trying to travel the wrong roads during my formative years. Thank God I finally saw it for what it was and dealt with it for what it was, sin. The more one avoids dealing with something, the more one becomes a prisoner of the past.

Don't be so pious, strong and mighty Christian. If you're thinking, "I sure am glad I've never been that bad off," you're missing the point entirely. We are all "that bad off." Jesus did not die just for my sins, but He died for the sins of the entire world. Romans 3:23 tells us, "For all have sinned, and come short of the glory of God." I neither have the time nor space to address all the sin for which Jesus came to die. However, the matter of suicide is a sin I have to address. I am not taking a stance as to whether or not one can get forgiveness for this mortal act, only that I feel it is in no situation any kind of answer or solution. It only creates more questions for those who are left behind. Any note left behind will never explain a suicide.

Do not be so brazen brothers and sisters in Christ; giants of the faith have also struggled with contemplating suicide. Maybe they did not as much as I have, but then again maybe more. My interpretation of scripture leads me to believe that the thought did at least cross their minds. Suicidal thoughts may not be a problem many people struggle with, but if this work can help one soul, it will have been well worth me sharing my hardship. Nobody other than God ever knows what is occurring in someone's mind. If the truth is never revealed, there may be more going on in your best friend's brain than you could ever imagine. Simply because we deny the existence of a thought in our mind does not mean it has never occurred. When I revealed my mental state to some of my closest friends, they were shocked. They could not believe I would ever even consider such a notion. Any red blooded American male can tell me he has never looked on a "hottie," as the kids now say, in lust, but that would only prove he will lie about other things.

Several men of the bible had the courage to share the personal demons they faced. King David, the man after God's own heart, had his moment of doubt in Psalm 55:6. In the depth of his depression he cried out, "...Oh that I had wings like a dove! For then would I fly away, and be at rest." The great writer Paul, who penned much of the New Testament, also had his moments of despair. In II Corinthians 1:8 he said, "For we would not, brethren, have you ignorant of our trouble which came to us in Asia, that we were pressed out of measure, above strength, insomuch that we despaired even of life...."

If you can't figure out what King David and Brother Paul were thinking, let me clarify their sentiments. They were tired of living in this world. Their words put it more elegantly than simply stating "I'm ready to blow my brains out," but that is how they felt. Alas, the prophet Jonah had just survived a near death experience when he had his moment of doubt and pain. After surviving in the belly of a great fish no less, he still begged in Jonah 4:3, "...O Lord, take, I beseech thee, my life from me; for it is better for me to die than to live." This man had just survived a near death experience to say the least. I can say I truly know how they felt. I am thankful I can stand in the company of such men, because in the end, they yielded to the Holy Spirit. Thank God they did not give in to the influence of the devil because we could hypothetically be without the beautiful book of Psalms, much of the New Testament, and 120,000 souls in the city of Nineveh would have perished. I want to emphasize hypothetically because Satan will never stop God's overall plan. God may have to find another one of His children to accomplish His task at hand, but the end result will always be God's will being done. These three men's words are simply a nice way to describe the nasty, secretive, swept under the rug, and whispered-only-in-closed-family-circles problem of suicide.

That was a big sentence for an even bigger problem. No one wants to confront it. No one wants to discuss. I know people who have committed this unanswerable act. I also know families who have lost a loved one because they were ambushed by this silent killer. And still nobody ever wants to open the door on this taboo topic for discussion. And no one certainly ever wants to admit he or she has ever entertained the thought of it. Well I have, and I am here to tell you about it. It, it, it. I am even referring to the act of suicide through the use of a pronoun now. It is as if I don't say suicide, suicide is really not around. Well suicide certainly is around, whether we talk about it or not, because suicide claimed the life of over 30,000 Americans last year. It is our eighth leading cause of death in America. Only traffic accidents exceed suicide as the cause of death among teenagers. Alas, between 1970 and 2000, suicide rates rose by 193 percent. The only place we want to see percentage increases like that is in our retirement accounts.

I like the analogy my mother gave me in reference to suicide. She told me, "you may not be able to stop the birds from flying over your head, but you can stop them from building a nest in your hair." I entertained thoughts of ending my life for too long before I sought help. This does not mean I wanted to act upon the thoughts, but rather that they kept returning. My doctors gave me the right antidepressants and a sleep aid. Soon I was feeling much better in regard to my mental state. After I got over the shock of my surgery, I was able to discontinue these two medications. I don't generally think we need to take drugs. However, there are certain cases, such as chemical imbalances, where they are helpful and necessary. Anytime the thought of suicide presents itself, it is a lie straight from the pits of hell. It is God's job to remove us from this planet, not ours. My writing has kept me busy during a difficult time in my life. While I was unable to return to work, I could still look forward to typing. It really gave me a sense of purpose and meaning. I'll now get off that soapbox.

After I stabilized in CVSICU, my doctors removed the various machines laboring for me. I needed to leave this support system in order to return to living on my own. The day after my operation I was out of bed, and my physical therapist had me walking around. I remember going to the operating room praying "Lord, whatever I must do to get back to life as I knew it, help me to wake up willing and able. No matter how bad I feel or how much I hurt, help me cooperate with my doctors and therapists to regain my strength." Even all the powerful drugs I took did not cause that prayer to fade. God kept the desire to recover and work hard at it burning fiercely in my heart and mind. A lot of people say "you were just lucky." To the contrary, I was just blessed. I don't believe in luck. I have RJR13 on my tag and got married on the only Friday the thirteenth in the year 2000 for a reason. It is because I am not superstitious.

I don't say this to be braggadocios, but the staff at Tallahassee Memorial Hospital remarked to my family that I was one of the best and most determined cardiovascular patients they had ever seen. This hospital ranks highly in the nation when it comes to heart surgery; they see a lot of patients, so I took that as a high compliment. Much of my recovery had to do with my age but not all of it. This kind of attitude is not a quality humans possess solely in and of themselves. It is of the Lord, a God-given fruit of the Spirit. Jesus warned Peter, in Mark 14:38, as He prayed in the garden, "The spirit truly is ready, but the flesh is weak." Then in I Corinthians 9:27 Paul tells us how he had to "bring it [his body] into subjection...". We all, as Christians, desire to do the right thing in life, but our flesh wants to do the exact opposite. While our spirit strives for the good, it must war with the sinful desire of the flesh to do that which is not beneficial. My mind was telling me to get out of that hospital bed and exercise, but my body did not want to hear it. Only the Lord can imbue you with the determination to get out of bed and walk when your flesh, possibly prompted by Satan himself, is pleading, begging, and screaming in your ears, "DON'T DO IT!!! LIE IN BED AND PULL THE COVERS UP OVER YOUR HEAD! THROW YOURSELF A PITY PARTY! THIS SHOULDN'T HAVE HAPPENED TO YOU! LIFE JUST ISN'T FAIR!"

Well guess what? Nobody, especially not God, ever promised anything about life being fair. For me to think this should not have happened to me for one minute is saying, "I am better than everybody else." Making that statement says my hardship should have fallen on someone else because I am too good to have it happen to me. Well I am not too good to face adversity, and neither is anyone else.

Eureka! Jesus didn't deserve to die on the cross. He didn't have to give His life as a sacrifice for sinners, yet He did because He knew there was no other atonement for mankind's sin. If He had thought, "I am too good for this," we would all be on the way to hell in a hand basket. Thank God for His humility.

In Matthew 5:45 Christ admonishes us to endure all things with a loving heart, "That ye may be the children of your father which is in heaven: for he maketh his sun to rise on the evil and on the good, and sendeth rain on the just and on the unjust." There is an old saying that goes the rain just so happens to fall on the just first, but this is not always the case. Bad things happen to good people, and good things happen to bad people. Also vice versa. God is no respecter of persons. We are all equal in His eyes meaning no matter how good people are, they are never so good to be above calamity. Some of the worst things I have ever seen in life didn't happen to murderers and rapists but rather to some of the Godliest people I have ever known. II Timothy 3:12 tells us, "Yea, and all that will live godly in Christ Jesus shall suffer persecution." It does not say might, probably, or could; it says shall. That means when we try to live for Christ, we can and should expect persecution.

Early persecution came in the form of being stoned, eaten by a lion, skinned alive, or dipped in boiling oil. These types of persecution ended rather quickly. I submit that Satan has simply changed tactics over the annals of time. Cancer, Alzheimer's, ALS, multiple sclerosis, muscular dystrophy, and manic depression these are to me the modern forms of persecution. If I had my choice, I would pick the lion over the cancer any day. The lion will kill in a matter of seconds or minutes whereas cancer can eat away at the body for months and sometimes even years. The mental afflictions seem to be the worst on my estimation because oftentimes the people afflicted do not even realize they have a problem until too late. Mental illness flies under the radar because there are usually no physical manifestations, only subtle signs that are easily overlooked by the untrained eye. This is why we see a happy, healthy, productive member of society one day and a corpse in the funeral home the next. Depression is easy to miss even in our closest friends. The people with the problem think it must be normal to feel like they do because they cannot "see" anyone else walking around who feels the same way. Also there is the stigma one faces with mental illness in our society of being labeled as crazy if one tells someone of one's troubles. Let's just say for the purpose of illustrating a point that I accidentally cut my arm off and I am bleeding to death. I am going straight to the doctor. If someone or everyone wants to label me one thing or another for getting medical attention, who cares; at least I didn't bleed to death. I know that is convoluted at best. I am simply trying to say we need not fear addressing and seeking help for any problem we face as human beings or Christians. It is a sad note that in the Christian community some of our own are afraid to ask for help because they do not want to be subjected to what others may say or think about them. The fear of what my family would think, coupled with the idea I could overcome it on my own, was one of the reasons I didn't immediately ask for help with my problem. This ought not to be so. We are to empathize with those suffering around us and help them in the best way we know how.

It gets hard to simply endure hardships sometimes let alone bear an infirmity with gladness and thanksgiving after the first few weeks, months, and what can turn into years. Only through the grace of God can a Christian bear any type of burden to His glory. Otherwise, you will become a bitter person, not a better person, because of your problems. We all get wake up calls at certain times in our lives. My dissection happened to me for a very distinct reason. God was telling me, "Time is shorter than you think son. It will expire on you one day, and it could happen before you ever know you are in the fourth quarter."

Once transferred to a private room, my rapid improvement continued. My family and friends aided in my speedy recovery at the hospital by visiting me to wish me well. I was so blessed to be surrounded by such a loving and supportive family and group of friends. I am eternally grateful for the patience they showed me. My wife was the best caregiver I could have asked for. And the nurses of Tallahassee Memorial Hospital are the best nurses in the world, in my humble estimation. I have been in hospitals all over the south eastern United States having tests run on myself or visiting loved ones. No staff even comes close to the "caring hands" philosophy exhibited at TMH. The nurses and doctors treated me as if I was their son or brother instead of just another cumbersome patient from a neighboring state.

Tallahassee Memorial Hospital has about four and a half miles of hallways. Unfortunately, I could only utilize a portion of this amazing length as my indoor track. Because of the transmission range of my heart monitor, I was restricted to the third floor. My nurses marked off all the places at which I had to stop. At the turn around points, I would beg Miranda, "Let me keep going so I'll drop off the monitor screen. I want to see if they come running and think I had a heart attack." No dice. Heart surgery does strange things to one's psyche. Mine was altered, and I don't know if it will ever be back to "normal" again. One immediate noticeable change was in my sense of humor. I now find morbid things funny whereas most people are repelled. The first good joke I got to play on people was April first. All day long when I saw anyone who knew I had heart surgery, I grabbed my chest and said, "I think I'm having a heart attack! Call 911!" After which I couldn't feign a pained look on my face but a few seconds before bursting into laughter. My friends and family failed to find the humor in that, especially my wife. Coming as close to death as I did will either make one laugh about it or cry. And I always say, "If I can't have fun, I ain't going!"

Miranda was so patient with me. She was always right by my side, in sickness and health, just as we promised each other in our wedding vows. We passed so many rooms where the patients had no loved ones in and out, no flowers or fruit baskets to brighten their days. They only had the great members on staff, but staff can only aid in recovery so much in regard to showing a patient love. Heart patients need the support of a family unit to give them support and encouragement. These key elements are vital components patients need to help them cope with the influx of foreign inner feelings. I do not know what I would have done without my loved ones' help and support. I do know I would not have bounced back as quickly as I did. Suffice to say, I am thankful I did not have to face my road to recovery alone. My wife and I did the best we could to brighten the day of my fellow heart patients with a warm smile, a kind hello, or a gentle nod of the head. I knew what they were facing, but not even that knowledge told me exactly what they stood in need of at any particular moment. Only God knew that. Even I didn't know what I wanted or needed to hear from time to time during my week long hospital stay.

The night before I was scheduled to be discharged, I awoke in an extreme state of confusion and panic. I had been dreaming I had not yet undergone surgery and was about to face it for the first time. I jumped out of bed, pulling out an IV in the process, and hurriedly shuffled to the bathroom mirror to see my scar and stitches for myself. I touched the thirteen-inch scar running down the center of my torso. As I felt the stitches on my fingers and saw the reflection in the mirror, I still thought I was dreaming. Even after I fully awoke, my brain couldn't believe that I had already had the operation. My wife had to reason with me and even had to page my nurse who had seen this all before, she explained. It was just a case of post traumatic stress. When one goes through traumatic situations, the brain oftentimes has a hard time dealing with it in the aftermath. After my discharge, my nocturnal confusion only seemed to worsen.

One night at home I rallied in the middle of the night to convince Miranda that the arm of the recliner I was sleeping in was actually the "arm of the recliner." I kept repeating, "I just don't think you really understand what you are looking at." It was like the arm of the chair kept insisting to me I needed to iterate its existence and purpose. It's hard to convince a sleep deprived heart patient that you really understand his point in the wee hours of the morning while maintaining a straight face. I'm sure it wasn't easy to do, but she convinced me I had gotten my point across and tucked me back into my Lazy Boy for more dreams of insane proportion. I awoke countless times in that first month following the surgery to talk nonsense out of my head and have no recollection of it the following morning. These nighttime diatribes became fodder for a good laugh over our breakfast the next day. My doctors said it was probably some lingering effect of the anesthesia I was under. I had a high dosage of some strong stuff because they kept me under for eight hours in deep sedation. Even now I dream about people whom I knew that have died on a routine basis. My cousin who is a psychologist told me that this is just a result of the rapid firing of neurons. I guess so...

Looking back, as I do a lot these days, I must have been in a mental state of shock while I was in the hospital. I can affirm that to know the strength of The Anchor, you have to feel the storm. It was three weeks or more after I came home that the reality of what I had weathered actually hit me. Dad was talking with a friend of his on the phone, who was inquiring about the procedure I underwent. I remember only getting half of a conversation to which I wanted to be the one asking the questions. Up to this point, no one had really, medically, explained my ordeal, and I hadn't asked about it because I was just glad it was behind me. I am sure my dad was still trying to accept that his only son had almost died. But I am a firm believer that you must know where you came from in order to know where you are. The only thing I still hold against my wife is the fact she failed to take any pictures of me immediately following the operation. They all said I looked "bad." I would like to be able to see how bad it really was. One afternoon a flying buddy of dad's called to check up on me and apparently inquire about what actually happened.

"Yeah Karl, they actually stopped his heart to repair the dissection. (Pause for Karl's side of the conversation.) This is the long and short of it. They hooked his body to a heart and lung bypass machine through an incision in his groin where they spliced into the femoral artery. This way they didn't have to clamp off individual organs, which is harder on the body and more time consuming. They were working with a limited amount of time. Once the heart and lung bypass machine was in place, his heart was stopped, thus eliminating the pressure on his aorta. (Pause for Karl's side.) The machine did the job of breathing as well as circulating the blood throughout his body. His body temperature had to be lowered to 59 degrees so there would be less risk of brain damage or stroke. {This is why I thought I was in a freezer just prior to the surgery. The thermostat in the operating room was set at 50 degrees.} Oh yeah, if he hadn't been at a controlled temperature, it would've killed him. The trauma his body was subjected to would have caused it to simply shut down on itself. The cold temperature slowed everything down so it took longer for his body to realize the damage that it was incurring. He was in a state of controlled hypothermia. (Pause for Karl's side.) {Also I am writing this now, so I suppose I incurred no more brain damage than I had prior to the surgery.}

"They were in such a hurry to get in there because they had no idea when the dissection would rupture. They said his aorta looked like ground chuck, so it was pretty close in their estimation. Like a matter of hours or minutes. If it had ruptured, the best trauma team in the world couldn't have saved him because too much blood would have been depleted from his vital organs. He would have gone into cardiac arrest. Each time his heart beat, he was getting closer to death. Once they got him on the heart and lung bypass machine, they had eliminated the threat of the pressure on the aorta. (Pause for Karl's side.)

"Then they had to run damage control. They outfitted him with a Dacron sleeve to replace his damaged aorta and a St. Jude mechanical valve to repair the bicuspid aortic valve. Both devices are cutting edge technology in heart repair they tell us. Years ago he would've died simply because this new technology wasn't around yet. (Pause for Karl's side.) Yes, Karl, he is a modern miracle. God still works through ordinary people to do extraordinary things. His surgeons were part of a miracle that day. (Pause for Karl one more time.) He's mending nicely now that he's getting to rest without being poked, pricked, and pressurized every hour. Keep him in your prayers as he is having a harder time mentally now, than physically. Thanks for calling. I'll tell him, talk to you later, pal."

I cannot comprehend or fathom my heart being stopped for eight hours while a machine kept me alive. Humor me. Can you even imagine how it would make you feel to know another person has touched your heart and actually stopped it, then cut away the diseased part, and replaced it with material like you can buy at the local hardware store? That is a rhetorical question, so I'll give you an idea; it makes me lightheaded, kind of like floating in the stratosphere to put it mildly. It was as if my life had reached its end, and God saw fit to give me a second chance. I thank God every day that He gives second chances and more. It makes no sense whatsoever to my logical mind because when your heart stops beating, you die. Generally speaking there are no exceptions. One has to think about this sort of life event abstractly, apart from any preconceived notion. That is the only way it can ever be absorbed. This is how I know that I am a miracle because by all logic I should be dead. When I pondered my ordeal, the journey in and out of surgery, confusion was the resounding answer I found in my mind. Medically speaking, my father has explained it to me countless times now, but I still cannot make rational sense of it. Time and time again, he has said to me, "Son, when they stopped your heart, they turned on the heart and lung bypass machine." Medical science has far surpassed my ability of comprehension. Knowing I have a piece of plastic in my body that keeps me alive is hard for me to think about. I can only imagine what a heart transplant recipient must feel like. I'm sure it is not easy to think about because I try to think about my mechanical valve as little as possible, but that is hard to do when I feel it and hear it with each beat of my heart. I have a clearly audible heartbeat. It sounds like a bass drum being struck every second.

I finally gave up on ever understanding, physically, what happened and how my body endured it on February 3, 2005. I say gave up when I should rather say I let go of the question. I have come to realize that what and how are not as important as why. I have learned to ask God daily, "Why am I still here today? Help me to discover what you want me to do today, and give me the wherewithal to accomplish it." I thank God every day for giving me a second chance to live. I praise Him for the miracle He performed in my life. I know Jesus healed the blind. I believe He fed the multitude. I have also seen Him heal incurable cancer with my own eyes. And when I experienced Him step into the fiery furnace with me, I knew without a doubt He had and still has

His hand upon me. He also brought me out of that furnace without so much as even the smell of smoke on me. That is when the reality of the situation took on an entirely different dimension. It is only human to question the how and why of experiences in life. Having time to distance myself from my ordeal has helped me understand questioning my fate is not a productive question. I simply give God the praise, glory, honor, and thanksgiving for the miracle which I am.

My life since the operation

I'm not going to lie. All my days have not been filled with bowls of cherries; some of them have contained nothing but the pits. However, I am glad to take the good with the bad. If we never had any bad times, how could we truly appreciate the good times? One of the hardest things I have faced has been getting accustomed to the sound of my artificial valve. Every time my heart beats, I hear a very noticeable thump. So loud it is that people near me can hear it as well. Just when I mentally get past thinking about my operation, this loud thump in the center of my chest reminds me, "You almost died." I suppose it is one way God helps me stay humble. I was sitting on the pew in front of a friend of mine at church one night. He asked me "do you hear that?" "No." Having grown accustomed to the "thump", I said "What are you talking about?" "It sounds like a kid is in the parking lot with their system blasting bass." Then it hit me that he was hearing my heartbeat. "No, that is my heart you hear beating." Michael thought that it sounded abnormal, "You better get that checked out shouldn't you?" "No, Mike I only have to worry if I don't hear that clear steady thump. That means I've got a blockage or a clot."

This sometimes makes me hesitant to go to quiet places where I will be in close proximity with people I do not know. When strangers notice it, they give me some funny looks. Now I just stare back and tell them if I'm not wound up every hour, I'll stop ticking. I know it's not funny, but sometimes I just can't help myself.

Another strange change in my body is that my sternum pops like my knuckles. Sometimes I just stand up, and it happens. Other times I twist my waist to make it happen. It relieves pain most times, but it also really disturbs my wife. I try not to do it often, but sometimes I just move the wrong way, and it pops. In conversation, it is always "since my surgery or before my surgery." It was as if time stopped on that fateful day and began anew for me.

I am also a lifetime member of the coumadin club. This means I am now a free bleeder. This has been a huge adjustment for me. An avid outdoors man, I used to cut and scratch myself routinely on everything imaginable. This especially concerns my wife when I use my chainsaw. If I ever got a bad cut, I could die before I got to the hospital. But I refuse to be an invalid. The way I see it, God didn't let me die on February 3rd for a reason. I will not be a hermit the rest of my life because I am afraid of dying. When my time is up, it will be up, and a bullet proof box won't save me from the inevitable. I simply must be extra cautious now because my blood clots very slowly. I have to check my protimes once a week to keep the viscosity of my blood within my doctor's acceptable range. This is tricky because everything I eat has an effect on my blood thinner. I have had a lot of trial and error in order to get to the consistency I am at now. This is the trouble with most people on coumadin. They are not consistent with their diet. My doctor wants me to stay between 2.5 and 3.5. In the beginning I used to freak out if I got too far off from 3.0, my mental goal. I have been as high as 4.8 and as low as 1.7, and nothing has happened to me yet. Coumadin will always fluctuate. That is something you just have to accept. I haven't had to stop living; I have just had to make changes in the way I live. For instance, if I cut myself shaving, it may take ten minutes for the nick to clot. I just take my time and don't get in a hurry.

The blood thinner, in addition to the blood pressure medicine, limits my physical exertion. Before surgery, I could work outside all day in the hot sun. Now a couple hours are all I can tolerate. If I push myself too much, I pay the price by feeling bad for a couple of days until I recuperate. I'm half the man I used to be. I just tell myself, "There is no need to try to do everything in one day. What will you do tomorrow if you get it all done today?"

Galvanic shock, the feeling one gets from touching a filling with a metal utensil, was an unpleasant phenomenon to deal with. When the chest is cut open, the nerves are cut right along with the skin, muscles, and tendons. This is no problem because they grow back together. However, it is slightly uncomfortable as they try to reconnect themselves. It feels like a small jolt of electricity every time they attempt to reconnect and miss their connection. As they all slowly grew back together, this pain completely stopped.

My bouts with depression still come and go. For the most part I keep my head up and just keep on living. Life has always been a journey for me, and if I stop, I'll never get to my final destination. Life is too short to stop by the wayside. There are too many more things I want to see, do, accomplish, and experience before it ends to waste a single minute feeling sorry for myself. When I do get depressed I look around because there is always someone who is worse off than I am. My wife is also good to give me a swift kick to the seat of my pants if I mope around too long. And that's a good thing to get sometimes. If you get depressed with your situation, go visit a pediatric burn unit, a cancer treatment facility, an orphanage, or better yet a Cardiovascular Intensive Care Unit. These places will certainly put you in direct contact with some people who are worse off than you are.

In conclusion, there is life after heart surgery. It is different than before, but in so many ways it is so much better. The air smells better to breathe. A flower is lovelier to look upon. A rib eye steak tastes better than it ever did before. Those old church hymns sound so beautiful they often bring tears to my eyes. And my wife's hand in mine, as we watch the sun set from our front porch swing, has never felt so wonderful.

Whatever we face in life, God is always only a prayer away. Our God is always as close as we want to be to Him. If there is any distance between us, it is a result of us, not Him. My advice is to not let sin tarnish a close personal relationship you can experience with God. Everything has already been said once and better than I could ever say it, so I'll close with a quote and go out strong. "Truth, like surgery, may hurt, but it cures." -Han Suyin

HE CAN WEATHER ANY STORM

My exercise in penmanship was supposed to end with the previous page, or so I thought. However, I would be amiss to exclude another miracle God performed in my life just forty-seven days after He so mercifully blessed me on February third.

March 22, 2005. I was taking my normal afternoon nap around 1:00. I awoke around 1:30, went to the restroom, and immediately fell back asleep. This was no problem because my body was still very weak from the operation, and I still wasn't sleeping well at night. Before I laid back down I glanced out the window to see it was lightly raining. The sparse drops were making small circular ripples on our pool. I remember thinking what a peaceful sight it was as I drifted off to slumberland. I had unknowingly just witnessed the calm before the storm. I awoke to my mother, much in the wet-setting hen fashion, who half dragged and half carried me into my hall closet.

She quickly packed pillows around me and covered me in several quilts in the closet to prepare for the worst case scenario.

911 usually alerts all the homes in Miller County of approaching severe weather by an automated calling system, but this time the storm struck too quickly. They say a tornado roars like a train, but from my personal experience I remember it whistling like a boiling tea pot sitting on a stove eye. This was not like the school house drills when we used to crouch under our desks and laugh at each other. It was the real deal. Mom knelt and anchored me as softly, yet firmly as she could to that closet floor. She also simultaneously began to pray directly from her heart to Jesus. Nothing fancy, pious, or liturgical, just five words were all she kept repeating, "Jesus please keep us safe." I lost track of how many times she whispered her prayer.

Having just awakened from a deep sleep I still had no idea what was happening outside. "John, we're taking a direct hit from a tornado. Whatever happens, keep your head down" she said. Immediately she was back to her plea to God. My mother does not get upset easily, so seeing her this way unhinged me to say the least. My emotions got the best of me for a moment. I remember thinking our house could be about to blow away in the maelstrom that was churning outside. Then I considered what God had just brought me through and how I had emerged unscathed. Instantly my fear dissipated. Jesus was right there with us as we kneeled in that hallway closet. We were calling on His name together, and Matthew 18:20 promises us that "where two or three are gathered together in my name, there I am in the midst of them." When Jesus makes a promise, it can be counted on.

I have experienced some bad weather, severe storms, and the outer bands of powerful hurricanes in our home. However, I have never seen any weather this bad or anywhere close to it and hope I never do again. I have formed my own opinion of what happened that terrifying afternoon. An atheistic meteorologist would no doubt argue with me over my conclusion. But the aforementioned did not sustain or shelter me during that tornado. God, His Son, and the Holy Spirit did keep me and my parents safe through the protection of their angelic servants. As quickly as the storm came, it passed on over. Nevertheless, I felt as if I lived out a lifetime in that closet. In reality, it was probably more like five to ten minutes. Fear can play tricks on your mind. Now back to my opinion.

God directed me to the 91st Psalm immediately after the storm passed. When my father gave the all clear, he told us he couldn't believe what he had just seen with his own eyes. "Come look at this. Ya'll aren't gonna believe it!" Doesn't that sound just like what any redneck would say? The view from the front porch was overwhelming. I asked, "Are you sure it's safe to be out of the closet yet?" We have a small sticker on our door with an angel wielding a sword that states, "Warning! This property protected by ANGELS WIRELESS SECURITY SYSTEM. Psalm 91:11-For he shall give his angels charge over thee, to keep thee in all thy ways." As I walked back into our home, I could not help but begin to think. I even glanced around outside half expecting to catch a glimpse of an angel sitting on the roof. I am not suggesting that tiny sticker offered any protection from the storm, but I know God's words did. God placed whatever number of angels He deemed necessary on and around my home that day. My limited and minute understanding of scripture leads me to believe it only takes one angel of the Lord, in His will, to defeat a legion of satanic forces. If you do not agree, opinions are like armpits; everybody's got one or two.

The street I live on had many 60 feet tall pine trees, some four feet in diameter, snapped in half. Massive 200-year-old oak trees were pushed up by the roots or pruned back to nothing but their stately trunks. One home completely vanished while several others were half carried away in the maelstrom. I am not trying to blow this account out of proportion, but this was a hellish storm. No pun intended. I have always heard we lived in "tornado alley," and now I know why this area is referred to as such. Before I get too far off on a rabbit trail, let me support my opinion of the angelic hedge which I briefly referenced. My application may be a stretch for some, so put on your spiritual thinking caps.

I have been told by men who possess Ph. D.'s that Satan is merely an imaginative farce to steer us to be morally good. I've also been told Ph. D. really stands for Piled High and Deep.... Intellectual learning can be a very valuable commodity as long as one never forgets who gave one the mind with which to learn. Unfortunately Satan is a real entity, very much alive and well in this present time. He knows his days are numbered by the hand of God Almighty. Therefore, he wants to do all the damage, cause all the pain, heartache, sickness, suffering, and sorrow he can before being cast into eternal hellfire. He may not fully realize or accept this as his doom, but I have read all of the Bible, and I know how the last chapter ends.

In the Gospel of John, Jesus warns us of Satan's aim for us. John 10:10 states, "The thief cometh not, but for to steal, and to kill, and to destroy: I am come that they might have life, and that they might have it more abundantly." The devastation we experienced in my neighborhood was not examples of abundant life, nor were they of Christ. It was destruction straight out of the pits of hell at the hands of Satan. Why God allows bad things to happen is an enigma neither I, nor anyone else, can solve. God's permissive will is a concept we will never fathom as human beings. Some things are simply beyond our comprehension. In Job 1:12 "the Lord said unto Satan, Behold all that he (Job) hath is in thy power; only upon himself put not forth thine hand." Not many verses later we learn of Satan's atmospheric control from a messenger informing Job, "there came a great wind from the wilderness, and smote the four corners of the house, and it fell upon the young men, and they are dead; and I only am escaped alone to tell thee" (Job 1:19). This verse proves Satan can use the atmosphere to do evil things to humans and even cause death if God permits it.

We know according to Ephesians 2:2 that Satan is "the prince of the power of the air" of the Earth. We live under this curse due to Adam's fall in the Garden of Eden. The Lord asked Satan in Job 1:7 "Whence comest thou?" Satan responded by saying, "From going to and fro in the earth, and walking up and down in it." Satan had been all over the Earth, just looking for something to stir up. I imagine his very presence and movements disrupt the area he inhabits. He is never happy. He cannot stay still, and he wants to hurt God and his children as much as he can. His toxic spirit tries to poison and disease all that he encounters. Satan is a highly intelligent being. He has been around since the world was created. However, he is very near-sighted in my estimation. John 12:31 refers to the devil as "the prince of this world." I could continue biblically proving how Satan has power presently, but that would be a waste of my time. I believe what the Word of God says in regard to Satan. He is alive and well in the world which we presently inhabit. He is a bad boy to say the least, and you do not want to tangle with him. If you are reading this and do not believe in Satan's existence, it is not my job to convince you he is real. That's God's work. I've done my part by planting the seed of God's holy, inspired, infallible, inherent word. Someone else will water, fertilize, and work the seed. However, as I Corinthians 3:7 reminds us lest we boast: "Neither is he that planteth anything, neither he that watereth; but God that giveth the increase."

That was a lot of information on Satan's power; however, it should not frighten a nonbeliever or especially a child of God. The Lord does not want us to live in a spirit of fear and bondage. Christ broke Satan's teeth out long ago when He gave His life on the cross. This is why the devil is called "a roaring lion" in Peter 5:8 rather than a biting lion. We have all heard the old saying "his bark is worse than his bite" used to describe a harmless yet noisy dog. This same maxim can be applied to our spiritual nemesis. He knows he does not have to bite us, just bark, and he gets to watch us shake in and of our own strength. This is why Christ warns in Ephesians 6:10-12 to "Be strong in the Lord, and in the power of his might. Put on the whole armour of God, that ye may be able to stand against the wiles of the devil. For we wrestle not against flesh and blood, but against principalities, against powers, against the rulers of darkness of this world, against spiritual wickedness in high places." Christ then instructs us to "take unto you the whole armour of God, that ye may be able to withstand the evil day, and having done all, to stand. Stand therefore…" (Ephesians 6:13, 14).

Twice, in back to back verses, Paul admonishes us to "put on" and "take unto you the whole armor of God." Once we have utilized God's armor, he further instructs us to stand. We are not to hide, retreat, cower, or posture in any other manner. If we do anything other than stand firm, it will result in ground given over to the enemy. That is the last thing a Christian wants or needs to do in a spiritual battle.

Thanks to C. I. Scofield's extensive research in the bible and revelation by our Lord, we have access to a plethora of pertinent information on our enemy. Footnotes from Revelation 20:10 reveal much in regard to Satan's powers and strength. "To him, under God, was committed upon Earth the power of death, he has access to God as the "accuser of the brethren" (Rev 12:10), and is permitted a certain power of sifting or testing the self-confident and carnal among believers (Job1:6-11; Luke 22:31, 32; I Corinthians 5:5; I Timothy 1:20), but this is a strictly permissive and limited power, and believers so sifted are kept in faith through the advocacy of Christ (Luke 22:31, 32; I John 2:1, note)." That is a long quote basically stating Satan can try us but only has the power to do what God permits him to do to us, most often due to our own pride or sinfulness. Luke 22:31, 32 paints a clear picture, "And the Lord said, Simon, Simon, behold, Satan hath desired to have you, that he may sift you as wheat: But I have prayed for thee, that thy faith fail not: and when thou art converted, strengthen thy brethren." The harvesters in times past would gather the wheat and continually toss it into the air to separate the fruit from the chaff. They only wanted the good part of the wheat to remain. The wind would blow the chaff away. Satan can and will sift us, but through our advocacy in Christ we, His fruit, will not be blown away. When all the sifting is done, all that is left is the good part, fruit of the Spirit.

I am getting around to paralleling my heart surgery with the tornado using Psalm 91. Some of the similarities are so ironic it is uncanny, but first back to the storm. When I came out of the closet and looked around, it appeared as if our small neighborhood had been under aerial attack. No pun intended. It literally looked like bombs had burst on trees, homes, and even places in the Earth itself. I had seen pictures on television of the scenes I witnessed that afternoon, but that kind of calamity had always happened somewhere else. Never did I think my friends, family, neighbors, or I would fall victim to such a disaster. Not that we wish misfortune or natural disasters on anyone, but it was like the cliché says, "one of those things that was not supposed to happen here." But just like my surgery, I am no better than anyone else to suffer loss.

Being an only child leaves my wife and me as the sole heirs to the family estate, not that we have a whole lot to inherit. What my parents have already turned over to us is an old, comfortable, sufficient, single-story, brick home which my Grandfather, built in 90 days by himself. That is another story for some other book. Two years after I married Miranda, my parents twisted our arms until we traded them our luxurious 56' x 14' mobile mansion for my childhood home. Three years of renovation later we almost had it like we wanted it when the heart/tornado trouble struck. Our mobile home, my parents' current abode, suffered extensive damage on each end. The two bedrooms took a beating due to trees pummeling them severely, yet we got off light compared to those in the surrounding area. My dad was about to go take a nap on his bed in the room that wound up with a pine tree top through it. It scares me to think what could have happened to him had he been in that bed. Thankfully mom convinced him to sleep in my recliner because she thought the weather looked rough outside.

Most homes on our street south of our house had to be covered in bright orange tarps thanks to the goodwill displayed by the fine folks at Home Depot. Props to that fine company as well as The American Red Cross, The Lions Club International, our local Dollar General, and Family Dollar. Yes, that was a shameless plug on my part. The hard work of F.E.M.A., G.E.M.A., Miller County Emergency Management Agency, Sheriff's Department, and Road Department employees will never be forgotten. In light of the Katrina disaster, lots of people poke fun at F.E.M.A., but unless you have ever lived through such a confusing event, you should not be so quick to point your finger. No electricity or telephones severely handicaps first responders during times of disaster. However, they are still out there putting their lives in jeopardy often for little or no pay. To be critical of such a selfless act is beyond unfair; it is down right wrong. Three Notch EMC, Grady EMC, Mastec, Musgrove, and Utilicon employees literally worked day and night until they restored our power on the 25th of March which was ironically enough, Good Friday. The Georgia State Patrol and Department of Transportation kept rubbernecks at bay during this time, and in doing so kept our street safe from further disaster by distracted onlookers. All our family and friends who helped us physically and financially during this time will always hold a special place in our hearts. If I have overlooked anyone here, I do apologize, but the outpouring of help and support was simply too much to keep track of. I simply say "Thank You!!!" once again. God sees all, and He knows all. What is done privately in this world will be one day rewarded openly, and God's rewards are far greater than my spoken or written praise could ever be.

Do not despair; I have another miracle to share. Other than downed trees all around our home, our dwelling place sustained no damage. The only thing even out of place on our house was the cap on top of the chimney. This was a miracle by nothing other than the hand of God. Not even a single shingle blew off our roof. As I said earlier, most of the other homes on our street had huge portions of the roof removed if not all of it. Why was our home spared? As my dad has always said to things he couldn't answer, "I can't answer that question."

Verse by verse I will now parallel the two miracles I witnessed at the hand of God. Soon after my surgery I claimed Psalm 118:17 to give me strength. It says, "I shall not die, but live, and declare the works of the Lord." With all I lived through in 2005, I saw plenty of God's works to declare, more than some people see in a lifetime. I continue to marvel at His wonderful work. Each morning He gives me the ability to get out of bed and see another beautiful sunrise. And I always think to myself, it is a great day to be alive! So as not to be repetitive, the following verses will come from Psalm 91:1-16 (KJV) unless otherwise noted.

Verse one states, "He that dwelleth in the secret place of the most High shall abide under the shadow of the Almighty." Here God promises if we will dwell in Him in His goodness and grace, He will "over shadow" us. If we will simply walk in fellowship with Him, He will shelter us through the storms of life. I'm having a good day today, but I do not know what you are facing at this time in your life. However, it is reassuring to know God is always there with us, in the good times as well as the bad times. He sheltered me from the moment I suffered my dissection, again during a perilous eight hour operation that could have killed me, and again through a severe tornado. What never ceases to amaze me is how God can take His word and through the Holy Spirit in us apply it to any situation He chooses. The Word is not limited to one single moment but is Living and able to transcend time throughout eternity. When David penned the 91st Psalm, he had no idea what an impact and effect it would have on my life thousands of years later. Each time I read the Bible, God is able to speak to me through a verse I may have already read countless times. That is why the Bible is often referred to as the Living Word of God. As with any living thing, it has the ability to meet any present need or situation.

In verse two David proclaims, "I will say of the Lord, He is my refuge and my fortress; my God: in him will I trust." This was my reality as I lay on a cold operating table waiting to be cut in half and as I huddled in a tiny closet during the tornado. There was nothing in this world to offer me refuge or protection other than my God and nothing I wanted to turn to other than Him. However, just verbalizing this belief is not enough. One must apply this faith on a daily basis. Faith cannot be in part but must be in whole. Not only can we say it, we must live it. With God it is all or nothing. There is no straddling the proverbial fence. When we try to hold on to control to areas of our life, we know God wants us to turn over to Him; He is not pleased. This selfish mentality grieves the very heart of God. Complete surrender to God's will and way is the path to complete freedom. Most people think they will lose control of their rights, but this is what the Lord desires. In giving God full reign we submit to His leadership and stop relying on ourselves. We all know we often make bad choices, but God has never made a faulty decision.

Being a slave to sin will never allow us any true freedom, joy, or peace. When we put our trust in anything other than Jesus, we will always fall short of God's desire for us. Wealth, health, fame, fortune, power, or possessions can all be swept away in the blink of an eye; a personal relationship with Jesus Christ can never be taken from us, even though we die. Christ is all we need, and all we should deeply long for if we ever want to be content in this present world. Wanting things just for the sake of having a lot of stuff will make us miserable people. Don't get it twisted; things are fine to possess. We just need to be careful to possess our things and not let our things possess us. Does my bass boat serve me or has it grown into something for which I live? Do I live my week with going out on the lake as my chief desire? We should never let things become the primary focus of our life. This is a truth lost people have a hard time understanding because the world tells them "he who dies with the most toys wins." And suffice to say, far too few Christians ever really comprehend and accept the freedom this concept brings. I've been to more funerals than I care to count, but there has been one common denominator at them all; I have yet to see a hearse pulling a U-Haul. The Hawaiians say "less is more," and there is a world of truth in those three little words.

The key to verse three, "Surely he shall deliver thee from the snare of the fowler, and the noisome pestilence," lies in understanding three definitions. First, a snare is a hidden trap or pitfall. This can be a man made, or spiritual trap. Do we still in modern times face snares? Just as surely as David faced these assaults, we do presently. Gossip disguised as a prayer group can snare some of the most well intentioned Christians. Satan will use these times of discussion to spread his agenda. "Did you hear about John? I heard he...." Pretty soon whatever befell Brother John was worse than it actually was and probably of his own doing. We should not try to make ourselves feel better than anyone who has fallen on hard times because if calamity hasn't struck you yet, just live long enough, and it will. It is not a fruit of the Spirit to kick anyone, lost or saved, while they are struggling in life. Most especially if they have entrusted you to pray about a problem, they have previously only had the courage to take to the Lord. If a people trust you enough to reveal something in confidence, do not break their trust by spreading their problem all over creation thinly disguised as a "prayer request." Individuals know when they are ready to share their need. We don't need to beat them to the punch by prefacing what they entrusted to us with "John told me so and so, but don't breath it to anybody." When people want their problems made public, they will announce it to the church themselves. It is our duty and election, as Christians, to put forth His attitude of humility. We should go to downtrodden souls to minister to them in genuine loving concern. This must start by building their trust, not breaking it.

The fowler is one who would do evil. The fowler is usually Satan or his minions but can be anyone who does not delight in the love and service of God. These people would rather exhibit the ways of the devil. If Satan can turn Christians against each other, I believe there is no greater thrill for him. He delights in sowing discord among God's children. He really takes no pleasure in how depraved a reprobate soul becomes because he has that soul where he wants it, lost with no hope in its salvation. However, if he can snare a Christian in one of his traps, it gives him reason to celebrate. When we sin and fall short of the glory of God, Satan says, "See. I told you so. They did it again God." This is why we need to truly turn our backs on sin when we repent of it. True repentance isn't just feeling sorry for sin but forsaking it all together. It grieves our Creator to see us trample on the shed blood of Christ repeatedly. Christ's atoning sacrifice does not give us a license to sin, just forgiveness for sin.

Lastly, the noisome pestilence can be likened to Satan himself. Noisome implies offensive, harmful, objectionable, disgusting, or injurious. Pestilence is a deadly disease or something that is morally or socially wrong. These two words describe Satan's agenda explicitly. What is so serious about all these big negative words is that they are camouflaged in the devil's tactics. He does not come out blowing the scent of fire and brimstone; instead he gently wafts the aroma of homemade cookies up our nostrils. He doesn't look like he does in the movies either because he can take on the form of an angel of light. He will not sound like fingernails on a chalkboard but rather like a well conducted orchestra. Not like a rough splinter in our finger will he feel but more like running the hand over a fine silk suit. Finally, his taste is not like sour milk. He will taste as sweet as honey while we swallow his lies hook, line, and sinker. Once we have bit on his "hook" is when he reveals the truth of himself. How true the old saying is that the devil is in the details. When he gives the thrill of that first time, he never allows one to see the devastation that is to follow. Only once the "hook" has been deeply set will one see the damage that is to come. He approaches us with the exact opposite of what he really is and what he has in store for anyone he can trip up. When something is too good to be true, it is usually not truth at all. This verse is relative to my situations in that Satan laid a trap to cost me my life by depriving my blood of the oxygen it needed to tell how sick I really was. Also he was no doubt in the noisome pestilence I experienced in the form of a tornado. However, God had His hand upon me through these troublesome times.

The fourth verse is a wonderful promise from God that declares "He shall cover thee with his feathers, and under his wings shalt thou trust: his truth shall be thy shield and buckler." This verse is the first scripture I remember reading after my operation. It was embroidered on a tapestry which hung in my hospital room and now hangs on our living room wall. The picture painted in my mind's eye by this verse is that of a mother eagle spreading her wings wide as she protects her offspring from harm. The eaglets trust in their mother so completely that they never doubt her protection. Their very existence depends on the strength, power, and commitment of their loving parent(s).

I submit that God is infinitely more compassionate than an eagle could ever hope to be. He has never once failed one of His children. He does, however, chasten the children He loves as any loving father should. He has a proven track record that spans history. It is difficult to trust someone whose character has not been proven, even more so to trust someone who has failed you in the past; but it only takes a little faith to trust in the awesome God we serve. He is able and He will as He has demonstrated from the Old Testament through the New Testament. God proves His love and faithfulness toward us each day. There is no need to doubt our Father who is so benevolent. God's truth is His Word, the Bible. It is His love letter to the entire human race. God is love and does not wish for any of His creation to suffer eternal separation from Him in hell. Nevertheless, there will be those who refuse to accept what the Bible says and repent of their sins. In doing so they will reject Christ's redemptive work on the cross, thus leaving God no alternative but to reward their decision with eternal hellfire. If you are reading this and have never been born again, you are lost, and your soul is in peril. Repent while there is still time. If you are not saved, turn to page 144 of this book, where I have recorded the plan of Salvation, and consider it now. Examine your heart. We never know when God's merciful hand will be withdrawn and we will enter into eternity. It could even happen before you finish reading this short book.

Verse four is a dear promise to me because of all the implications it holds in regard to my two separate situations. First, during my surgery, a machine kept my body alive for eight hours. My heart was stopped so it could be repaired. When your heart stops, your soul is supposed to exit its earthly tent. I have struggled with what happened to my soul during this short time. As I have said, I saw no bright light at the end of a tunnel. There appeared no angels or demons while I was under the anesthesia, nothing good or bad. All I remember was the anesthesiologist telling me, "Everything is going to be all right. Just breath deep for me and this will be over before you know it." God sheltered my body from physical harm just as He protected my soul from spiritual departure. During the tornado, God kept me safe during a storm that produced winds in excess of 200 miles per hour. I know this because it blew down power line structures that were engineered to withstand 200 mile per hour winds. Belongings from a neighboring home were found in a town that is 90 miles away. My life and home were spared by God's hand and His hedge of angelic protection.

The miracles I saw first hand still make me scratch my head in awe. Why did God see fit to spare my life, not once but twice? Survivors' guilt is a phenomenon that most people who have a close encounter with death will face at some point after they realize how close they came to dying. For some people this thought just crosses their minds briefly, but for others it can develop into a debilitating disorder. I have stood by the gravesides of several of my own peer group and watched as their caskets were lowered into the ground. In my estimation they were all too young to die. Why didn't God intervene in their lives as He did in mine? My first intimate friend I lost to death, Bruce Anthony Williams, was killed in a car wreck on the night of his eighteenth birthday. He is the person who is directly responsible for introducing me to my wife. I was only nineteen when Bruce died. I had and still have a hard time believing I will never see him again on this Earth. The accident happened ten years ago this year, and it still sometimes feels like we just left the graveside. Not a day goes by that he doesn't come into my mind for one reason or another. And even now as I pen these lines, I am still mourning the loss of a dear childhood friend, Justin Calhoun. He was a young man with the rest of his life ahead of him. To me, he was cut down in the prime of his life. He was a loyal, courteous, kind, and gentle soul who always wore a smile on his face. It was the kind of smile that was contagious. When you were around him, you left feeling better than when you arrived, even when things were not going his way. I saw him endure a medical device I would liken to medieval torture. The halo he wore positioned screws through his skin directly into his bone; no doubt it was a painful contraption to say the least. Yet when visiting him, I never heard him complaining. He just smiled through his pain and proclaimed how blessed he was that it had not been any worse. Justin may have been short in stature, but he was a spiritual giant to me. Why did he die and not me? Why were sixteen others I can name off the top of my head not given the second chance I was afforded? The short answer is that their time on Earth was up, and mine was not yet. This is where the speculation must end, or we can wind up in a place where we spiritually do not need to be. It is not our place to question God's timing. People die, and to those left behind it will never happen at a good time. I don't know anyone who has not experienced the loss of a loved one. There is no way to sugar coat this cold hard fact of life. If we live long enough, we will all discover that the old saying is true, "two things you can count on are death and taxes."

God wants us to be open and honest with Him. We cannot hide our true feelings even if we try. However, we need not fear expressing our grief or inability to understand tragedy. Christ promises us in Matthew 5:4 that "Blessed are they that mourn: for they shall be comforted." When I am hurting, I want and need comfort. I can think of no better healer than Christ.

Times of sorrow and loss are when we must whole heartedly exercise our faith in God's authority and decisions. It is far easier to accept being overlooked for a promotion than it is to accept your wife is going to die from cancer. We must be careful not to blame God because He is not the reason sin entered into this world. It is mankind's own doing at the temptation of Satan. If we had all the solutions to life's unanswerable questions, pretty soon we would try to put ourselves on the throne in God's rightful place.

I was deep in thought, trying to wrap my mind around these feelings of guilt for being alive, when I realized who I needed to call. A highly educated Christian psychologist put this in perspective for me one Saturday morning as I was still recovering from my surgery. He is a decorated veteran of the Vietnam War. He flew in 187 combat missions over hostile territory. He lost many comrades and fellow aviators in the war in Vietnam. Remarkably, his plane never got a single bullet hole in it on all those perilous missions. Was that mere chance? No, it was divine intervention. He has dealt with far more survivors' guilt than I have for many more years. He knows and understands this guilt well. His words of wisdom to me were "our Father was not ready for us yet. He still has a purpose for us on this Earth." Another veteran, who received a purple heart and still has a bullet lodged within inches of his aorta, echoed the same sentiments. He has also had heart surgery so he understands my situation very well. When random people are telling you that you are alive for a reason, it is reassuring, but when some one who has gone through the same peril you have and worse says it, the words really take root.

Comfort and strength are drawn from verses five and six as we are told "Thou shalt not be afraid for the terror by night; nor for the arrow that flieth by day(5); nor for the pestilence that walketh in darkness; nor for the destruction that wasteth at noonday"(6). It is not God's will for us to go through life in a state of constant paranoia. Nor does God want us to be scared in regard to any particular situation or obstacle in life. As long as I can remember, my Dad has always told me, "life is a serious undertaking son, and nobody is gonna get out of this world alive."

Apart from being translated in the rapture, we will all eventually face death. I do not fear death; I just don't like to think about the grief it will cause my family. When our eternal destination is secure, we have nothing to fear. This is why the thought of dying has never bothered me. I accepted Jesus at the age of five, and for those of you who are wondering, yes, I knew exactly what I was doing. I will never forget announcing to Mom that I wanted Jesus to save me and live in my heart. She explained the plan of Salvation to me, and I knew God was convicting my young heart. As I knelt in front of an inexpensive, red, vinyl couch at my Dad's car lot, God changed me from His enemy into His child. I was instantly made a new creature through the finished redemptive work of Christ on the cross. He saved me and sealed me. Suffice to say, I have always known whose I was and where I was going. When we found my bicuspid valve at the age of eleven, I always seemed to sense

Memoirs from my Mended Heart

heart surgery was on the horizon for me in some shape or form, and it has long since been my worst fear. Some kids my age had nightmares of Freddy Kruger or Jason, but I awoke terrified a doctor was taking my heart out of my chest. I never even told my wife or parents about this until after the surgery because they think I am dramatic enough as it is. Carrying that kind of fearful energy and emotion around will eventually affect one's attitude and life whether one thinks it will or not. I am here to tell you from first hand experience. I now see that a lot of the problems I faced were a direct result of trying to handle this apprehension on my terms when I should have simply turned my fear over to God who can handle any and all problems. Not trusting God to solve our problems and meet our needs will take us down paths we do not need to tread. No matter what we face, God knew we would face it before we were ever knit in our mother's womb. Psalms 139: 16 says "Thine eyes did see my substance, yet being unperfect; and in thy book all my members were written, which in continuance were fashioned, when as yet there was none of them." God knew all our faults and flaws, physically speaking, before we were ever even formed In our mother's womb. He made provisions to sustain us physically, spiritually, mentally, and emotionally through any and all situations in life, even our worst fear. Given and entrusted to God, our fears become a non issue. You're probably thinking, "That's easy for you to say." It is because I have lived through it and testify that this statement is true. God has kept me safe through some frightening times in my past, but the ordeal that unfolded on February 3 was my worst fear realized. It also struck out of nowhere. I went to the hospital looking to come home with some high powered pills, a shot in the worst case scenario. Instead I was told, "John, this problem is going to require immediate invasive surgery in order for you to live." In cases of most bypasses and even valve replacement the doctors usually have the luxury of time on their side so they can schedule the surgery at your convenience. This was not so in the case of my dissection. I had no time to prepare mentally. It was just a bomb of bad news that hit me like a nuclear warhead. Looking back, I'm thankful it happened the way it did because I never really had time to get scared or fearful because I was still in shock that this was happening to me. God always knows what He's doing. Some people may be brave enough to arrive for an open heart surgery appointment at six A.M.; I would have probably skipped the country.

Terror, arrows, pestilence, and destruction are certainly things we can attribute to the devil. He wants us to live in a constant state of fear, doubt, and confusion. His desire is the exact opposite of God's will for our lives. He is a liar, the father of lies, and attempts to counterfeit all that God does. Sometimes his traps are easy to spot, and other times we must exercise careful discernment to see his camouflaged snares. Terror was what I initially felt as the doctors told me I had to undergo surgery and as I was crouched in the closet during the tornado. It was nothing I did to rid myself of this feeling. Philippians 4:7 references this other worldly serenity by promising, "And the peace of God, which passeth all understanding, shall keep your hearts and minds through Christ Jesus." Humans cannot pull this pacific quality out of their mental faculties. We certainly cannot muster it in their soul. However, God can and will grant us this wonderful gift as we rely on and trust Him in life.

I compare the arrows to Satan's "fiery darts." God's word promises us His "shield of faith" will stop these satanic attacks. This is going to be a real spiritual stretch for some, maybe most; this theory could have been born due to the lack of oxygen to my brain for an extended period of time. I believe Satan literally tried to kill me by assaulting my spiritual breastplate and my physical sternum. He literally unleashed hell on my heart and watched to see what would happen next. Satan had no way of knowing the miracle God was working in my life through his plan of ruin and destruction. God took all the evil Satan threw at me, and He used it for good. God allowed the surgeons to repair my dissected aorta, my bicuspid valve, and then rejoin my severed sternum with titanium. Now my sternum is stronger than before because it is bone and a super light space age alloy. This may be another stretch, but I also think Satan thought he could kill me by inflicting intolerable pain and suffering upon my body. Human beings are medically only supposed to be able to tolerate so trauma before their body simply gives up the ghost. Yet even in the worst pain I ever want to experience, I never even passed out. I came very close though.

Satan delights in death because it causes humans unimaginable pain. I have a much deeper respect and understanding for Christ's suffering on the cross now than I did before my operation. When Christ died on the cross, Satan thought he had won. He probably started himself a little party here on Earth during the three days before Jesus arose from the tomb. Satan actually thought he had succeeded in killing the Christ of glory. He was no doubt stupefied when Christ regained His life on the third day and later in Revelation 1:18 boldly proclaimed, "I am he that liveth, and was dead; behold, I am alive for evermore, Amen; and have the keys of hell and death." In Ephesians 4:8 we learn that during the time in between His death and resurrection Christ "led captivity captive, and gave gifts unto men." Christ's work during this three day hiatus from Earth also afforded the Apostle Paul the spiritual strength, in I Corinthians 15:55-57, to pen "O death, where is thy sting? O grave, where is thy victory? The sting of death is sin; and the strength of sin is the law. But thanks be to God, which giveth us the victory through our Lord Christ Jesus." Christ pulled the stinger out of the bumble bee of death. He defeated the grave and our earthly battle against it. He broke the law's authority over us when He paid the price of our sin for which we were to be judged. Therefore, He afforded us the final victory.

These trials in spiritual and health related battles did nothing to weaken my spiritual breastplate; they only served to strengthen it. Just as my sternum was strengthened, my walk in the Christian faith was also made stronger in the Lord. Satanic attacks can come in many different shapes and forms. Satan will attack us spiritually, mentally, emotionally, physically, and these four areas are just his starting grounds. He just gets warmed up on this stuff. He knows our weak spot(s) and believe you me, we all have them. We have to keep our guards up at all times and stand strong in the Lord, never trusting in self. Trusting in our own strength will get us nowhere but tripped up, flat on our face eating dirt, because Proverbs 16:18 teaches, "Pride goeth before destruction, and a haughty spirit before a fall." God looks at the attitude of the heart. We would do well to apply God's standard in I Samuel 16:7 "...Look not on his countenance, or on the height of his stature; because I have refused him: for the Lord seeth not as man seeth; for man looketh on the outward appearance, but the Lord looketh on the heart." When we display a judgmental attitude, we need to remember we all have a soul, and God looks at our hearts, not our bank accounts, social status, or physical appearance. He does not judge us by our "filthy rags" because we all are lacking in the light of His glory. He sees us through our relationship in Christ, and in Him we are righteous before a holy and just God. We also learn of our saintly status in Ephesians 2:19, "Now therefore ye are no more strangers and foreigners, but fellowcitizens with the saints, and of the household of God." This means we share more than a passing similarity with the saints of God It tells us we are saints of God. This is and always will be heady for me, but it is easier to accept God's deep spiritual truths than to question them.

Pestilence and destruction can be examined together because they are very much one and the same. These words both share negative connotations. They are not qualities of God. Once again, we know Satan desires only to "seek, kill, and destroy," proving he wants the exact opposite of Christ's desire for us to have abundant life. Christ wants us to live to bring glory to His Father, but Satan wants us to die so we can no longer give God any glory or point lost souls to Jesus. I find it very interesting that live spelled backwards is evil. This is a prime example of how Satan turns the words of God around, literally. Live is what God wants us to do while evil is what Satan wants to do to us, and how he wants us to behave so that we grieve our Maker. Many people don't understand this and go through life trying to determine why they have so many problems. Proverbs is full of real life applications. In Proverbs 14:12 we find another one, "There is a way that seemeth right unto a man, but the end thereof are the ways of death." We often think we are on the right path, yet at the end of our way we discover we were sadly mistaken.

Actively seeking to live for Christ will in no way ensure you an easy life. Quite the contrary, a life of submission will make your days much harder than going your own way. However, you will have the calming assurance of knowing where your problems are coming from and why Satan is throwing them your way. As Brother Jeff Robinson once told me, "Any dead fish can float down stream; it takes a live fish to swim upstream." It boggles my mind how God can use negative situations and evil to bring about good in and through our lives. Without my heart problem you wouldn't be reading this now. I would like to think some good will come of the effort I have put into this little book. Maybe I'm not being too presumptuous. Just as Satan uses the negative for evil, God comes along and uses it to strengthen us and help us live fuller, more productive lives for Him.

It is no small coincidence that verse six states "the destruction that wasteth at noonday." When I learned I had a dissection and when the tornado hit, it was just after twelve o'clock, noon. That was destruction attempting to waste me at noonday. The diagnosis could have been pronounced at nine o'clock, and the tornado could have struck at six o'clock. But they did not. They occurred, I believe, the way they did to prove God's infinite wisdom to me. God knew when the 91st Psalm was written that it would have a great application in my life many, many years later. That just blows my hair back every time I think about it! Some people may think I am crazy, or laugh me off as a fanatic, but when you love someone or something, you are going to be passionate about them or it. And I love Jesus Christ and His Holy Word. They are my true passion and purpose in this life. Everything else pales in comparison to seeking daily to find and do God's will in my Christian walk.

The Bible goes on in verse seven and eight to state "A thousand shall fall at thy side, and ten thousand at thy right hand; but it shall not come nigh thee.(7) Only with thine eyes shalt thou behold the reward of the wicked.(8)" Let me emphatically state I am not saying anyone in this world is a wicked person because this or that does or does not happen to him or her. All I can judge is me, and I hope I am harsher on myself than God is going to be. Why good people die each year from aortic dissections and in tornados, I cannot explain. In the words of my father, "I can't answer that question." I simply must accept that it is part of God's plan for this world, His ability to bring good from a seemingly bad situation. There are certain situations we will never understand this side of eternity. One day we will see "face to face" and have the "mind of Christ." Precisely why God chose to heal me and protect me remains a mystery to me. I did not deserve His mercy and grace. Lots of times now I feel even more undeserving of His blessings than I did in the past. I think this stems from the fact that I know I am now closer to the Lord than I have ever been before. After all, that should be our goal; to daily draw closer to our Lord and Savior. I used to think I actually deserved for God to be good to me. I suppose this could be a reason God used my ordeals to humble me and bring me to my knees. I thank Him daily for the miracle He performed in my life.

Why do bad things happen to good people? I'm just going to throw this out there to be considered. I have an idea that in the end Satan's judgment will result in a courtroom like showdown. In Luke 21:13 Christ tells of coming hardships, and then He states "And it shall turn to you for a testimony." Also in Matthew 18:18 He promises us "…Whatsoever ye shall bind on earth shall be bound in heaven: and whatsoever ye shall loose on earth shall be loosed in heaven." This tells me that the things we do and endure while on this Earth will come back into play in eternity. Picture this: God will be on His throne with Satan still arguing his case. Satan's pride will lead him to make a final attempt to dethrone God. He really thinks and believes he can prove that sin should be acceptable to God. That is the worst part about pride; the arrogance, megalomania, and delusions of grandeur that come along with it. All these characteristics rolled up into one being make quite a nasty fellow. Keep in mind he has been hard at work honing his skills for thousands of years. In our earthly courtrooms, the defense must call witnesses to prove their case. God doesn't have to adhere to our protocol, but I feel he will so that He can once and for all prove to Satan that his offenses are inexcusable. He will call His "witnesses" to discount Satan's accusations. Satan will be convicted before all of creation, and if he continues to argue after the sentencing, there will be no one to listen in the bottomless pit. Even though we know a criminal is guilty in our legal system, evidence still has to be presented against the perpetrator. When I say God's "witnesses," I mean people we see as having gotten a raw deal in their life on Earth. We often think of them as having died before their time in our mortal minds. The devil should have learned by this point not to argue with the Most High, but he will prove to be rebellious to the very end. Satan's allegations and claims will be obliterated by the testimony of God's own children. Form your own opinion; that's just the way I see it.

Now why did I live when others my age died? What was God trying to help me see or learn? I have clearly seen that God's ways are so much higher than our ways. Psalm 139:6 says "Such knowledge is too wonderful for me; it is high, I cannot attain unto it." This is the bottom line when it comes to God's ways. No matter how much we study His word or strive to understand Him, we will always fall terribly short. That is just another fact of life. Nevertheless, we are to follow Paul's admonishment found in II Timothy 2:15 where he encourages Christians to "Study to show thyself approved unto God, a workman that needeth not to be ashamed, rightly dividing the word of truth." We are to try to walk as close to God as we can, but our sin will always be a barrier to ever perfectly communing with Him while on Earth. Even if we don't commit sin during the day, we omit doing things we know we should. We must confess our sins to God each day before we will ever be close to where He wants us to be, spiritually speaking. When we make it to the point of spiritual maturity God wants, He will give us our next assignment, eternity. We can't get a diploma from a school until we learn all that the teachers require us to know. And so it is with our God. When I die, God will in effect be telling me I have learned all this life has to teach me.

My faith in Christ's ability to heal me and my submission to His will is what kept me from an early grave. If I had attempted to tell God what to do, or tried to bargain with Him in regard to my life, I don't believe I would be here today. "You've got to fix me. I'm too young to die." That was not my prayer, but rather, "Lord, not my will, but thine." That was the prayer of Christ in His most difficult hour. He did not want to drink that bitter cup, but more importantly he wanted His Father's will to be done. And just as I argued with my earthly father to not go to the doctor, he knew, better than I, what was best for me. Doing the will of the Father is a difficult point to come to in life. It requires much spiritual discipline. It took so much effort on Christ's behalf that He actually sweat drops of blood, a medical condition brought on by an unbearable amount of stress. I didn't sweat blood, but I was no doubt wigging out. We must not only do God's will in the big things but in the small details of life as well. Do we do His will when no one is around to see us? That is when we are who we truly are.

Verse nine and ten reveal a cause and effect relationship: "Because thy hast made the Lord, which is my refuge, even the Most High, thy habitation; there shall no evil befall thee, neither shall any plague come nigh thy dwelling." God is my refuge, not my insurance policy or my bank account. Because He is my refuge, He did not allow anything bad to happen to either of my dwellings. Neither my body, nor my house was damaged in either incident. He is my refuge in the good times and the bad times because I put my trust in Him alone. For God to be our refuge and habitation, one of the most relevant factors is self-denial. This is a daily process, not a one time event. This is the hardest part in regard to presenting ourselves as a living sacrifice. Without the grace and strength of God, a "living" sacrifice will crawl off of the altar. Verse nine points out our duty and responsibility to God while verse ten shows us God's promise to us. If we put our refuge in anything other than God, we will be sorely disappointed to say the least. We must make our relationship with God our top priority in life. If we do not, we tarnish our fellowship with Him and grieve the Holy Spirit. I have tried to fathom events for which there are no explanations in life for quite some time now. One Grandfather died when I was three, the other when I was five. That was 25 years ago, and I am no closer to understanding why it happened now than I was at five years old. It is only human to analyze things we cannot comprehend. God made us with minds that are finite for a reason. I believe it is so that we must rely on Him fully and completely. If God gave us all the answers to all the mysteries of life, who would we go to for wisdom and understanding? Our learning can only come from God. Books are good, but man's teaching can never compare to the greatest teaching that that is of God. His Holy Word is the first book we should turn to in life, especially concerning problems, questions, and solutions we face or need in life. Everything we can or will ever face has already been addressed in the Bible, by God, the original self-help author. So many times I run to the Christian bookstore for a self-help book where all I need to go to is my Bible. Are you guilty of the same, friend? The Christian bookstore is a wonderful resource and complement to God's Holy Word. However, it should never be a first resort but rather a supplement for our walk through life.

As I stated before, bad things do happen to good people. Some of the worst things I have ever seen in life have happened to some of the best people I have ever known. Why? I can't answer that question as dad says. I can only speculate that God knows who can handle what. Therefore, He allows the cream of the crop to suffer the worst because they become such great examples of the faith to those of us who are not so mature or strong. And God is attentive. Nothing ever catches Him unaware. He knows the number of hairs on our heads. Have you ever watched the dust in a gyre through the sunlight pouring in a window? Not one speck of dust in the air settles to the floor that He does not know where it will end up. He also cares for the birds of the air. Meditate for five minutes on how much more He must love His creation for whom He sent His only Son to die on the cross.

God sends the rain on the just and the unjust. Job was a man who understood adversity in a biblical sense. No pun intended. He will always be remembered for his patience and humility. He was a godly man who had bad things befall him, and he was still able to say with conviction in Job 1:21,22, "Naked came I out of my mother's womb, and naked shall I return thither: the Lord gave and the Lord hath taken away; blessed be the name of the Lord. In all this Job sinned not, nor charged God foolishly." When we arrive at the point where Job was, we will be where God wants us for times of trial and tribulation. Most people go through their entire lives and never come close to the spiritual plateau of Job. Only through serious trials and tribulation have we ever had our patience refined the way Job's was. When someone says, "John Doe's got the patience of Job," it is because he has been tested and tried, and he came out true. So be careful when you pray for patience because I only know one way to get it, the hard way. James 1:3 says "that the trying of your faith worketh patience." So utilize the patience God has already given before you pray for more. When we are squeezed in the vice of life, what is really inside will come out.

I have made numerous references to the existence of angels. If you doubt me, here is my promise from God to support me, o ye of little faith. Verses eleven and twelve contain two powerful promises, "For He shall give His angels charge over thee, to keep thee in all thy ways. They shall bear thee up in their hands, lest thou dash thy foot against a stone." I know in my heart of hearts I was surrounded by angels the day of my operation. I also know my home was protected by them during the tornado. I can offer no concrete proof, but my faith points me to this conclusion. Our society has commercialized angels to the point of desensitization; much as it has with Easter and Christmas, but that's another book for another time. Highway to Heaven was one of the first mainstream media introductions to angels. It was a great program. Then along came Touched by an Angel, another good show, but they never mentioned Christ. They only referred to God in broad, general terms. Hebrews 13:2 states "Be not forgetful to entertain strangers: for thereby some have entertained angels unawares." On a lighter note, do you know where in the Bible it says the man makes the coffee? He-Brews! That is one of my favorite corny jokes. A country song made reference to this verse, but they never sang about the Christ the angels serve. Angels are wonderful as well as references to them, but we never need to emphasize them more than God, who created them.

With that in mind here are some thoughts I have on the angel of the Lord. These two verses are not symbolic. They are literal. God knows Satan's moves before he ever makes them; therefore, all He has to do is send one of His angels in His name, and Satan's plan is instantly ruined. Situations we encounter in our day to day lives are not a random chain of events. Nothing in life happens by luck or chance. Circumstances are formed by the very hand of God for a purpose that we may never be fully aware of until we get to heaven. Then we will understand everything we have gone through while there were no answers in this life. I imagine we may even discover the reason we had that flat tire the morning we were already late for work. All our questions will become crystal clear.

God actually uses His angels to protect us in our everyday lives. The Bible bears out this fact. Elijah was fed by an angel as Jezebel pursued his life. When Satan tempted Christ in Matthew four with all the kingdoms of the world, angels came and ministered to Him after He had successfully resisted the temptation. Also before the crucifixion Christ was strengthened by an angel. In Luke 22: 42,43 we see Christ having His moment of weakness just as we do; "Saying, Father, if thou be willing, remove this cup from me; nevertheless not my will, but thine, be done. And there appeared an angel unto him from heaven, strengthening him." Christ overcame His moment of doubt and fear by relying on the power of God and focusing on His mission here on Earth. Apart from this same attitude we will never overcome anything in our lives, especially our weaknesses, fears, or doubts. Satan knows exactly what they are and how to use them against us. However, calling upon the Lord will bring us all the power we need to defeat our foe in all the battles of life. I feel He even sends His unseen servants to do battle on our behalf when the struggles of life warrant it. God grants us His grace in many different ways, and He promises in James 4:6 that "he giveth more grace." This is one of my favorite verves in the Bible because one portion of grace should be enough, but God says he will give us more grace when we need it. That is the epitome of beauty in my opinion.

Christ even asked God to remove the cup of His wrath from Him, if it be His will, but He ultimately wanted the Father's will to be done. This is how we must pray if we want to develop a Christ-like attitude. We must accept God's will for our lives even if it's not what we necessarily want. Moments of doubt and fear will come because we are only human. Yet we must submit to our Father's will, as Christ did, to bring Him His rightful honor and glory. It is wonderful to serve the true and living God. He is acquainted with all the trials and tribulations we will ever face in this life. He is not a dead prophet who was simply a good man. Christ is the God-man. God said it, and that settles it. God the Father, Christ the Son, and the Holy Spirit are the true and living God. They are one being, and each is a separate Deity. Our minds have a hard time understanding that, but it is a fact. To accept that fact is much easier than attempting to prove God wrong. Christ is not only acquainted with our petty problems, but much more than we will ever endure in this life. None of us will be despised and rejected the way He was. We will never die the death He died on the cross. Even if we do suffer dying on a cross, we will not carry the sins of the entire creation on our shoulders. Now, back to the angels...

An angel came to Joseph and Mary, each separately, before Christ was ever born. Joseph was warned to flee by an angel so that Herod would not kill Christ in His infancy. Christ no doubt had angels at His disposal as He matured into a man. As Jesus was arrested in the garden, He reminded Peter He could call down more than twelve legions of angels, or 72,000 if He chose to do so. As He hung on the cross all He had to do was say the word, and legions of angels would have been at His immediate defense to save His life. However, Christ had a greater purpose in mind as He hung on that cruel cross, you and me: "And being found in fashion as a man, he humbled himself, and became obedient unto death, even the death of the cross" (Philippians 2:8). Our savior had angels at His service, and He still uses them to do His bidding in our modern day society. As my Mother has always said, "times may change John, but God never does." Angels do not sit around on clouds strumming harps all day. No, they do God's will tirelessly, thwarting the devil's plans. It will be such an honor to be one day counted among God's eternal heirs.

In verse thirteen we learn what we can do to Satan through the power of Jesus Christ: "Thou shalt tread upon the Lion and adder: the young lion and dragon shalt thou trample under feet." God granted me victory in my trial of heart surgery. He also gave me the provision to weather a devastating tornado that ravaged my community. No insurance policies are as good as the promises of God. They will all fall short no matter how much they cover. We are in the best hands to ever be in when we are in God's hands. Satan has power in this world, no doubt. However, his power against believers is strictly limited to the permissive will of God. Once we accept our gift of Salvation, we are sanctified and sealed, safe in the hands of our Father. No matter what Satan throws our way, none of his attempts to harm a Christian will work if God doesn't allow It to happen. However, trusting in self, money, a job, health, worldly knowledge, or anything other than the Lord will lead down the wide path rather than the straight and narrow. All material things in life are temporal. They are for us to use to serve God in the here and now. Things were never intended to bring us joy, satisfaction, or purpose in life. In Luke 12:34 Christ teaches us "for where your treasure is, there will your heart be also." This is why it behooves us to loosely hold the things of this world in our hands. Material possessions can disappear as quickly as they appear. This is a fact too few people realize until a calamity falls upon them. If we lay up our treasures on Earth, moths and rust can corrupt them, or thieves can break a lock to steal them. Service to our Lord with our time, talent, and tithes will always be secure in Heaven. I lived a life of self-fulfillment for many years. I am acquainted with the emptiness it produces. Nothing good ever comes from always putting our wants and desires before God's will. True freedom and joy only come through surrendering our rights to God. If we hold on to our rights, they will possibly be violated. However, if we resign our rights, they cannot be stepped on because we will have turned them over to God. If we go around concentrating on ourselves, our rights will be forever intruded upon or abused.

Happiness found in material possessions is a lie of the devil. It is a cheap counterfeit of the true joy God will give us if we seek Him first. Even the physical realm of life cannot bring one fulfillment because that which is born of the flesh, and not of the Spirit, is born to die. Eventually, even the most healthy, beautiful, or handsome body will break down and begin the process of decay. This is a result of the curse we live under. But one day for the Christian, "This corruptible shall have put on incorruption, and this mortal shall have put on immortality, then shall be brought to pass the saying that is written, death is swallowed up in victory. O death, where is thy sting? O grave, where is thy victory? The sting of death is sin; and the strength of sin is the law. But thanks be to God, which giveth us victory through our Lord Jesus Christ." I Corinthians 15:54-57 are verses I hold dear to my heart, thus the reason they are repeated here. However, we cannot take one verse and base our life upon it. We must take the Bible as a whole to understand God and His plan for us.

The next verse, fourteen, is powerful scripture: "Because he hath set his love upon me, therefore will I deliver him: I will set him on high, because he hath known my name." Once we are saved, God records our name in the Lamb's book of Life. Some people have a hard time with my wife's name. Just for the record, it is Miranda, pronounced Muh-ran –da, like the Miranda rights. Anyway, people call her Amanda, Mandy, Melissa, or they butcher the spelling on our Christmas cards. This is the point. All like to hear their name and to hear it pronounced correctly. I am certain our heavenly Father has no problem with her name because He has it written in the Lamb's Book of Life. I guess that is just a pet peeve of mine. Being called by the wrong name makes one feel unimportant or overlooked. In order for God to record our names in the Lamb's Book of Life, He had to send His only begotten Son to pay the debt for our sin, once and for all. Some of the good ole boys where I come from down here in the South would lay down their life for their prize hog hunting dog, heck maybe even their wife. As I stated earlier, my sense of humor has been warped. My parents would lay down their life for me. I have always believed that when they told me, but I came to fully appreciate on April 24th, 2007 at 11:29 A.M. when our son John Anthony "Hines" Roberts was born. The moment I saw him if someone would have told me it's either you or him, I would have said well it's gonna be me. And I will harbor that same sentiment for as long as I live. Possibly some "true blue" friends may seriously consider dying for one of their best friends. However, I don't know of anyone who would die for a complete stranger who is going to curse them after they die. Christ tells us in John 15:13 that "Greater love hath no man than to lay down his life for his friends." I am thankful Christ saw me as His friend.

There are five people I would give my life for without even thinking about it; Jesus Christ, Miranda, Hines, Sue, or Bob Roberts. Why? These individuals would reciprocate in the same manner if circumstance required it. As a point of fact, Christ already died for me so I could spend eternity with Him. The three aforementioned humans, excluding my son, have all done more for me and given me more love than I ever deserved, much as Christ did. My son has done nothing for me yet other than make me the happiest man alive, so he qualifies without saying. Yet Christ came to die for the whole world, fully knowing many would reject His gift of unmerited favor and love. Our mortal minds cannot comprehend dying for someone who does not love us in turn. That love, agape love, must come from a pure, undefiled, holy heart. The only heart like that ever to inhabit this world was the heart of Christ. We as simple humans are not capable of mustering such will power or such a show of determination. Show me a man who is willing to suffer and die the death of a cross for his enemies, and I'll show you a man who should seek psychological attention. However, Jesus Christ suffering and dying on the cross of Calvary shows me the heart and passion of God's only son. He is the Savior, who became the propitiation for your sin and mine. He bled and died for us while we were enemies of His Father. And why? Because from time immortal, God knew there would be a need for mankind's redemption. He looked out across eternity and saw the greater good that would come from Christ's death. I often ask myself, "Self, when is the last time you sacrificed yourself for your King?" and if I am honest with myself, the answer is never. I do my best to do God's will, but I have never had to actually sacrifice for Him. Witnessing to a lost person is about as close to sacrificing as most of us will ever get. But how much of a sacrifice is it to share the greatest news in history? It takes a little of our time, a little of our courage, and a little of our commitment. It's really not that hard. It's a joy and a privilege as well as our responsibility as a Christian to spread the good news of Salvation until Christ makes His imminent return. Only upon His return will God's overall plan of Salvation be complete.

God promises to set us apart or to "set us on high" because we know and recognize the name of His Son Jesus Christ. The Bible teaches in Acts 4:12 that "Neither is there salvation in any other; for there is none other name under heaven given among men, wherby we must be saved." Once we are saved, through the name of Jesus, God holds us tightly in His grip. There is nothing Satan or man can do to harm us. Love, honor, glory, and praise are what God deserves from us. It is what is due to Him, not only because He has proven himself faithful, just, righteous, and holy which He has time and time again, but simply because He is the great I Am. God deserves our love and devotion because He is the true and living God. When one factors in the tremendous unmerited favor He shows us, it should only multiply our thanksgiving and loyalty to our master.

Speaking of loyalty, I have a pit bull. She has to be the most loyal breed of dog I have ever owned. Wherever I am, whatever I am doing, Maggie wants to be right there next to me. If she is loose in the yard and I am working outside our fence, she will climb over the fence to make her way to her master's side. I scold her to stay in the yard. I tempt her with treats left in her house. I even got a chain link kennel to put her in, and she chewed through it. She has even cut her belly badly in some of her fence climbing. In short, there is no end to this dog's devotion and loyalty to me, her master.

It makes a good illustration of how we should feel toward Christ. We should be willing to do whatever it takes to stay clean and close to our Master's side, even in the face of any and all opposition. Persecution, temptation, imprisonment none of these things or anything else should stop us from getting as close as we possibly can to Jesus. After all, the only reason I am still living and breathing right now is God's matchless grace. And without His mercy I would be doomed and damned to a devil's hell. That is what we have earned and what we deserve, but glory to God He sees things differently. He sees things in a light that would blind us. He says we deserve the abundant life, joy unspeakable, and peace that passeth all understanding here and now. Even better than that, He says we deserve eternal life, eternal joy, and a perfect body with which we will spend eternity serving Him. And all we must do is reach out and accept His Son as our Savior. So why do people want to make salvation so complicated? Is it a lack of faith? Is it a hard heart? Is it the love of self more than the love of God? Could it be pride? I don't think there is one definitive answer to the question. Those questions were merely posed to get you thinking.

There are many different reasons people reject Christ. However, they all have one thing in common. They will all be inexcusable in the final judgment. There is no justifiable reason for rejecting Christ in the final analysis. Any reason one gives for rejection will ultimately drag one down to Hell. I encourage, no sternly implore you, let go of whatever is keeping your heart from accepting Christ and run from it as fast as possible. Accept Christ as your personal Savior before it is too late. I am proof positive that we never get to plan the day we will die. When I woke up on February 3rd, I had no idea I would face the possibility of entering eternity. Yet face it I did. Death is a sneaky thing because for us, there is never really a convenient or good time to die is there? Nevertheless, whether we are prepared or not, we will all one day enter eternity. Do not miss heaven. I have heard it said that most people miss heaven by a mere 18 inches, the distance from the heart to the brain. Don't try to reason or rationalize; just search your heart. God and His Holy Spirit will do the rest because He does not want any of His creation to end up in Hell. Sadly enough though we know many will find it as their final destination. God established the plan of Salvation so that even a small child can understand it. When we accept His Son, He will in turn accept us, even with all our faults and flaws. I don't wash my car before I take it to the car wash to get it cleaned, and so it is with our coming to Jesus.

All 16 verses of Psalm 91 are wonderful promises of God. The next verse, 15, promises "He shall call upon me, and I will answer him: I will be with him in trouble; I will deliver him, and I will honor him." Calling upon God does not result in an audible answer, at least not for me. In Genesis 3: 8 God spoke directly to Adam. The Bible says, "And they heard the voice of the Lord God walking in the garden in the cool of the day...." It is hard for me to imagine what it must be like to actually talk one-on-one with the creator of the universe as Adam did in the beginning of history as we know it. I am sure it must have been a wonderful conversation to say the least. However, once we enter the New Testament, His voice is heard less and less with the ears. In Matthew 17: 5 God directly addresses Peter, James, and John while in the company of Jesus. Peter was talking with Christ as He was transfigured, and "While he yet spake, behold, a bright cloud overshadowed them: and behold a voice out of the cloud, which said, This is my Son, in whom I am well pleased; hear ye him." Again, when Jesus was baptized, the voice of God was heard in Luke 3: 22. "And the Holy Ghost descended in a bodily shape like a dove upon him, and a voice came from heaven, which said, Thou art my beloved Son; in thee I am well pleased."

I believe our spirit "hears" the voice of the Lord through His written word, and the Holy Spirit bears witness with our spirit to affirm the word of God. Presently if we tell lost people we "heard God speak," we would get some strange looks and maybe even be considered by some to be mentally unstable. To this end, God speaks to us through His Holy Word in which we find the words of His Son. I suppose talk shows may help thousands of people each day. Some of them even rush home to get advice on a certain issue or problem. However, when a Christian has a dilemma or crisis, we need go no further than the pages of the nearest Bible. Most of our problems develop because we only open our Bible when we get into a quagmire rather than depending on the Bible for direction every day. Thank God He is always faithful. He never moves one inch on His throne. No matter how far we stray, or how long we stay, our Father is always watching and waiting with open arms for our return. I am reminded of the father who waited day after day for the return of his son in the Gospel of Luke. If we will only humble ourselves, we can enjoy sweet communion with Him anytime. The toughest trial I have ever faced to date was heart surgery. In my darkest hour God held my hand tighter than I ever remember it being held. I still struggle with the why of what I went through, but I heard a wise minister once say, "No where in the Bible does God ever promise to explain, but He does promise to sustain." And sustain us He does.

I have had many questions since my ordeal. I have often wondered why I had this happen to me and why I came so close to dying but lived to tell my story. Thankfully, I have an awesome support system in my wife, parents, family (physical and church), as well as my close friends. Many people are not so blessed.

Thank you to you all. You know who you are. One of my cousins, a minister and educated psychologist, told me "it is a lot easier to accept the unfathomable mysteries of God rather than try to rationalize them." I have come to find that statement to be very true. When we think we understand God, it puts Him in a box, and we limit Him in our mind. God knows my heart, and the last thing I would ever want to do is put a limit on Him. Even a direct answer from God in regard to our mind-boggling questions will not ease our pain. It would only lead to more questions which would quickly become extremely problematic. For instance, if God told me, "John, you suffered an aortic dissection because you were born with a weak aorta," my immediate response would be, "Why did you create me with a weak aorta when I could've had a perfect one?" On and on the questions would go because no answer would likely satisfy. I would be chasing the proverbial rabbit trail to nowhere. This is a slippery slope best avoided by simply having faith and trusting that God knows exactly what He is doing even when we cannot comprehend or see the purpose of a seemingly bad situation. Even when we can't see His ultimate plan, we can still trust His hand. What we need to cry out for in hard times are not answers, but rather strength and direction.

What I have tried to do with this work is give God the honor and glory for the miracles He has performed in my life. This is what I should have been doing all along since the day He performed the miracle of saving my wretched soul. But just like my dear Brother Paul had to learn in Acts 9:5, "it is hard for thee to kick against the pricks." In times past, herders used poles with sharpened ends, commonly called pricks, to make animals go where they wanted them to go. Sometimes the livestock didn't want to go there, so they kicked at the pricks, thus inflicting undue pain and torment because ultimately they were going to wind up in a greener pasture whether they wanted to or not. So it is with us. God gently nudges us in the direction He wants us to go and when we don't respond He may resort to "pricking" us, physically or spiritually. When we are not obedient to His will, we cause ourselves anguish that would be best avoided. Life is hard enough without creating undue trials and tribulations. Each day will bring us all the problems we can handle without seeking to help God in perfecting our patience by creating our own set of problems to face. I know I am not where I need to be spiritually. Spiritual growth is or should be a lifelong process culminating in our heavenly homecoming. When one can face being devoured by a lion as the early church did, I feel spiritual maturity has been reached. This is the point God wants all of His children to reach eventually. It just takes some of us longer than others.

At the end of verse 15, God promises, "I will honor him." Webster defines honor as "public distinction for a worthy symbol or worthy of respect." This is my heart's deepest desire, to enter the portals of glory and hear my Father say, (this is in South Georgia speak), "John, you have done us proud ole boy. Now I in turn have something for you; eternal life with me. Well done thy good and faithful servant: enter into the joy of thy Lord. You fought a good fight, you finished your course, you kept the faith!" If we honor God above all else, He will in turn give us our heart's desires. And if we are honoring God above all, our desires will be in line with His will. If we fail to give God His proper place in our life, we sell ourselves short of the countless blessings He has compiled for us, just waiting to bestow on His faithful and obedient children. Don't get this twisted. We do not serve Him in expectation of blessings. We serve out of love and in order to become more Christ-like. We are blessed as a result of serving out of a pure heart. Christ entered this world giving of himself to serve others, and He died a death of service so that we may have forgiveness of our sins, no self-gain or ulterior motive, just pure, unadulterated love. Once we ever fathom the depth of Christ's love, we will never be the same.

Finally we reach the last verse of the 91st Psalm. God promises to honor His children in verse 16, "With long life will I satisfy him, and shew him my salvation." We all want to live, not die. However, whether we live to ten or one hundred, any length of time is insignificant in the light of eternity. I have come to understand that it is quality, not quantity, which matters when it comes to living life. I would rather live a short life which is close to Christ than to never even touch the hem of His garment, though I live to be the oldest man since Methuselah. If we will only try to draw near to Jesus, He has so much more for us than simply touching the hem of His garment. One of my favorite verses, James 1:17, speaks of His blessings. It teaches, "Every good gift and every perfect gift is from above, and cometh down from the Father of Lights, with whom is no variableness, neither shadow of turning." I love that. It is so poetic and descriptive. I can see God in my mind's eye, never changing, never wavering; He always does what is righteous and just.

In the days of old when the stone workers would build an archway, there was one stone called the keystone which carried the weight of all the other stones in the arch. The keystone had to fit perfectly, or the arch would collapse. I thought the carver would fashion the stone up near the gap in the arch. This was an incorrect assumption. I have learned the carver was so skilled and experienced at shaping stone that he only had to look at the void to see just what he needed to cut away to make the keystone fit. From the image he saw in his mind, he set about chiseling away the rough edges of the keystone while at ground level; an inch here, a centimeter there, and then a huge chunk on one side of the stone. Only when the process of shaping the stone was complete would he hoist the heavy centerpiece up to its final lofty resting place. This was the process because once the keystone was set in place, it would have required much effort to take it down and hoist it up again. The stone worker had to get it right the first time to avoid an undue amount of work. To me, this is how I think God uses this world to shape His children for eternity.

Some of us fit into eternity with little shaping required. We all know Christians who we see as giants of the faith, people we look up to and often turn to in rough times for spiritual guidance. Others, like me, require years of shaping. It may take a sledge hammer, an extremely sharp chisel, and possibly a stick or two of dynamite to remove the unnecessary "stone." I was a huge boulder, figuratively speaking, and I had a lot of excess stone that God knew needed to be removed while I was still at ground level or here in this life. The excess stone I am referring to are things like pride, selfishness, hate, greed, envy, gossiping, and lots of other sins; the list could go on. Since my birth, God, the Master shaper, has been busy chiseling away, continually removing the rough edges. He will continue to shape me until I am finished and prepared to fit into the "keystone gap of eternity."

A child is born with the sin nature. As we grow in age we become more polluted by the things we see, say, and do in this world. This pollution can only be washed away by the blood of Jesus. I have always been of the opinion that life is a test, not a beach. We are tested everyday whether we realize it or not, and God sees our reactions to situations that befall us. He watches how we react to the "little" problems in this world to see if we are ready to handle the "big" responsibilities of eternity. We must be faithful and true before we are ready to enter eternity. The only way I know to prove our sincerity to God is to live in such a manner that we are willing to do the right thing, even when there is nobody around to see us other than God.

Being faithful and true, boy is that a tall order. Many times my parents have placed me in a position of responsibility because they trusted me. Oftentimes I did the right thing, but sometimes I did not. Sometimes I got caught by them, and sometimes I did not. Either way, I always knew in my heart when I had not done the right thing, and my conscience ate at me. My mom also usually instinctively knew when I was involved in wrong doing because a mother just always knows. She always forgave me but would tell me "you have broken my trust. Now you have to earn it again." That statement has taught me much about God over the years since my childhood. Mother's suspicion always faded, and she would eventually trust me again even if it was after a period of parentally imposed probation. Some of my friends said I stayed on pp (parental probation) from pre-school right up to graduation from high school.

All jokes aside, I am glad God doesn't place us on probation when we sin. The only probation is self-imposed by not confessing and repenting of our sin to restore a right relationship with Him. God continues to give me chance after chance. I am so thankful I was born in the dispensation of grace rather than in Old Testament times because I would have likely ended up dead. II Peter 3:8-10 is as comforting as it is fearful: "But, beloved, be not ignorant of this one thing, that one day is with the Lord as a thousand years, and a thousand years as one day. The Lord is not slack concerning his promise, as some men count slackness; but is longsuffering to us-ward, not willing that any should perish, but that all should come to repentance. But the day of the Lord will come as a thief in the night; in which the heavens shall pass away with a great noise, and the elements shall melt with fervent heat, the Earth also and the works that are therein shall be burned up." One day, and it will be sooner than we think, our lives on this Earth will become a vapor. We will be here one minute and gone the next.

This writing has been very cathartic and therapeutic during my recovery, as I was told it would be. I have wanted to write a book for as long as I can remember. Being a published author has always been one of my goals in life. I just never could nail down something that would be compelling, interesting, and beneficial enough to put on paper. After my surgery, I began a journal, and I quickly saw that I was on to something. God gets glory more than any other time, I believe, when lost souls are saved. That is the ulterior motive that compelled me to write this book. If one person accepts Christ as a result of reading this, it will all be worth it because a soul is intrinsically valuable, and it can't have a price placed on it. In the scripture from II Peter we learn the bottom line. God sees time through the lens of eternity. He desires that all of mankind would be saved. However, He is holy and just; He cannot lie. Therefore, there will be some poor souls who are caught unprepared and will suffer the eternal consequences of their lack of preparation.

Back in the "good old days," my dad grew up two tenths of a mile from where I presently live. His parents neither locked a door at night nor window for that matter. Now, all across America we have to nail down all that we own, or it may not be there in the morning. Even then, our property sometimes still turns up missing. Times, or rather people, sure have changed over the years. I have that pit bull who is bad to the bone and would probably die in my defense if need be. I am also a staunch believer in my right to keep and bear arms. My point is that, we must be prepared for situations that arise unexpectedly. I keep my property secure. My dogs let me know if a stranger is trespassing. Therefore, I can and will defend my family if need be, God forbid. I said all that to say this. When a thief or murderer shows up, there is no time to go procure a watch dog and train him or buy a gun. You better have your preparations made and know what you are going to do because in that situation, as dad says, "it's all over with except for the crying son." "Be prepared" is the Boy Scout motto. On a fellow Eagle Scout's first camping trip I really learned a valuable lesson. The forecast called foe lots of sun. The forecast was wrong. Josh was the greenest scout on the trip, but he was also the only camper to stay dry as it rained non stop the entire weekend. He packed a poncho while the rest of the troop neglected to bring this important piece of gear. On all camping trips afterwards, I never got caught out in the rain because of Josh's lesson.

So it will be with the return of Christ the King, all over but the crying. But wait friend, you do not have to shed a tear. Repent while there is still time, and you can cry tears of joy rather than sorrow. God's merciful grace has given you the time to read this short book. Get your relationship with Him secured through Jesus. Bow your knee to Him while you have a choice, and there is still time. One day the time of choice will be lost, and you will bow and acknowledge Him as King of Kings and Lord of Lords whether you want to or not. Do not wait until God's precious gift of eternal life with Him is unattainable. I implore you, beg you, accept Christ as your personal Savior, and enjoy a life with a relationship with Him. There is no greater decision you will ever make in this life. One of my Christian mentors, Brother James Ursrey, always reminded me, "We need to stay packed up and prayed up because we never know when we are going to go up."

I recorded my thoughts and feelings in these pages because the human experience is meant to be shared. Being on the introverted side, sharing these words with people, possibly some I never even met, has been challenging. Being a human, not to mention an only child, sharing is not something that comes naturally to me. But thank God, He's still working on me. We are all selfish by nature. We want to satisfy our desires before we even begin to think of other people's needs. However, the Christian living in God's will flips the script. Born-again believers seek to please God first, others second, and somewhere down the line they may begin to think of themselves. What joy is it to go through life putting yourself before all else? I submit that there is no true joy in that lifestyle at all because I lived that life for many years. It is only full of isolation, misery, and emptiness of the spirit.

Collecting my thoughts has been very beneficial to me. It has given me comfort, hope, joy, and peace in the midnight hours when I could find no rest. Rather than wallowing in my misery, self-pity, tossing and turning in bed, or counting sheep, I kept hearing a familiar voice in my mind telling me to write. "Get up John. Write it all down, for there is coming a time to rest. It is simply not here yet." I still experience times in the night when I have difficulty sleeping. And I have a saying I now use when my wife or parents question my sleep patterns. "I can rest when I die." They usually are quick to change the subject. The days immediately following my operation were the worst and best in my life. Never before have I hurt so badly, physically, but more so emotionally. On the other hand, never have I felt so loved by God and the loved ones who surrounded me. God's hand was and is very clearly upon my life. I will never regret taking the time to write this book, regardless of what may come of it. It is but a small part of the legacy the Lord has blessed me to leave behind one day.

As dad eventually says when we go up flying, "It's time to bring it in for a landing." That said, I will offer these short comments in closing. If you ever feel like an elephant is standing on your chest, get to a hospital even if it feels like he steps off. Our body was created to warn us when something is wrong. Do not ignore clear warning signs like I foolishly did. It is better to err on the side of caution. When you fall on hard times in life- if you haven't yet, you will- focus on other's rather than self. Taking note of others problems always seemed to make my personal issues seem petty. That will surely give you a clear picture of people with worse problems than your own. If you are depressed or suicidal, talk to a spouse, parents, pastor, or an intimate friend about how you feel. There are physiological symptoms to depression, as well as mental. Do not let a problem get out of control that can be addressed and treated. If the depression warrants it, go see a trained mental health professional. Above all else, talk to the Great Physician through Christ. After all, who can cheer the heart like Jesus? Nobody cheers the heart like Jesus. A loving support system is vital, but Christ at its head is imperative. It is my hope and prayer that these words have encouraged a mended heart and soul in some small way. If not, I warned you what was to come on the first page. And if my words did not help you, they sure did make me feel better to get them out of me, and that is what I needed at this particular point in my life.

Post Script

The Christian life is all about serving others, and through this act of selflessness we find ultimate joy and freedom. Only in the Lord will we ever find complete fulfillment. Christ summons us in Matthew 11:28-30: "Come unto me all ye that labour and are heavy laden, and I will give you rest. Take my yoke upon you, and learn of me; for I am meek and lowly in heart: and ye shall find rest unto your souls. For my yoke is easy, and my burden is light."

The only true rest we will ever find comes from Christ. The only yoke we will ever enjoy wearing is the yoke fashioned by Christ. The only burden that will ever feel light is the burden Christ gives us the strength to shoulder. The path I have been on since February 3rd, 2005, has not been a walk in the park by any means, but neither has it been unbearable. This is due to my Lord and Savior. He has given me much needed rest, insight, as well as support when I was at my weakest.

As I write these final pages, it is 4:30 in the morning. I awakened from a dead sleep really scared and not knowing why. There has been a lot of that kind of stuff since my surgery, an overwhelming sense of panic for no plausible reason that goes away after no more than a few seconds or minutes. But while I'm freaked out it usually feels like I'm about to die. At least that is what my mind is screaming. It will be five months to the day since I came out of the fog of anesthesia in one and a half hours. I will die believing that, every time I awake around this time on the anniversary of my operation, something clicked in my brain that I will never be able turn off. It is like an internal alarm clock that always goes off on the fourth of each month. But rather than hearing the radio, I hear "Get up John. Get going, for the time is getting short." There is no medical evidence to support my theory, but there are so many idiosyncrasies that come with heart surgery I do not think the medical professionals will ever document them all.

I do know that every patient's experience has its similarities, but no two are exactly the same. I think above all else my mind is still playing tricks on me this early in my return to normalcy. It is still hard to understand how eight hours can become so life-altering. My best advice to anyone who is about to undergo or has recently undergone heart surgery is to get saved if you are not, and get solidly grounded in the Word of God. That is just good walking around advice anyway because we have no idea when our time is going to be up. And once we stand before God, there is no turning back.

Before my surgery I was a Christian but a very ineffective one at best. God has a reason and purpose for every soul on this planet. I failed to see the magnitude of actively seeking and doing the will of God. I was happy with the status quo, simply sitting and soaking, failing to share my faith outside the doors of my church. That is exactly what Satan wants. He doesn't mind Christians going to church, but he doesn't want them inviting any of his crowd to sit under the Gospel. I am no longer happy with the status quo. I thought going to church was enough to let everyone know I was a Christian and they needed to be saved. I want to take Jesus out the door with me and share Him with a lost and dying world. Christ teaches us that a life of obedience, faithfulness, love, purity, and service is what He wants from us. That may seem extreme to some, but He took extreme measures so that we could inherit eternal life.

As I said at the end of the first section, I once heard that everything's already been said once and better than I could ever say it, so I'll close with a quote and go out strong. "You never know how much a horse will pull until you hook him up to a heavy load." -Paul "Bear" Bryant

Plan of Salvation

"For all have sinned, and come short of the glory of God."
Romans 3:23

"For the wages of sin is death; but the gift of God is eternal life through Jesus Christ our Lord."
Romans 6:23

"But God commendeth his love toward us, in that, while we were yet sinners, Christ died for us."
Romans 5:8

"But what saith it? The word is nigh thee, even in thy mouth, and in thy heart; that is, the word of faith, which we preach; That if thy shalt confess with thy mouth the Lord Jesus, and shalt believe in thine heart that God raised him from the dead, thou shalt be saved. For with the heart man believeth unto righteousness; and with the mouth confession is made unto salvation."
Romans 10:8-10

"For whosoever shall call upon the name of the Lord shall be saved."
Romans 10:13

It is as easy as A,B,C.

Ask.
Believe.
Confess.

finis

Special Thanks
Miranda E. Roberts

I could have never done this without you, baby. Your servant's heart and strength of character encourage me more than you will ever know. You did not let me give up, and you never let me keep the mullygrubs for long. You gave me a reason to fight to live, and you will always have my love and devotion simply because of who you are. I love you.

"Who can find a virtuous woman? For her price is far above rubies." (Proverbs 31:10)

God, my Heavenly Father, Christ, my Lord and Savior, and the Holy Spirit, my Comforter: Eternal thanksgiving is yours. You all did so much for me before I even had a chance or tried to do anything for you. I will praise you because you are worthy. I will declare your love, works, and truth because there is nothing greater in this life.

"The Lord hath appeared of old unto me, saying, Yea I have loved thee with an everlasting love:

therefore with loving kindness have I drawn thee." (Jeremiah 31:3)